THE

BHAGAVAD GITA

TALKS BETWEEN
THE SOUL AND GOD

THE

BHAGAVAD GITA

TALKS BETWEEN
THE SOUL AND GOD

translated from the Sanskrit with commentary by

RANCHOR PRIME

with illustrations by
CHARLES NEWINGTON

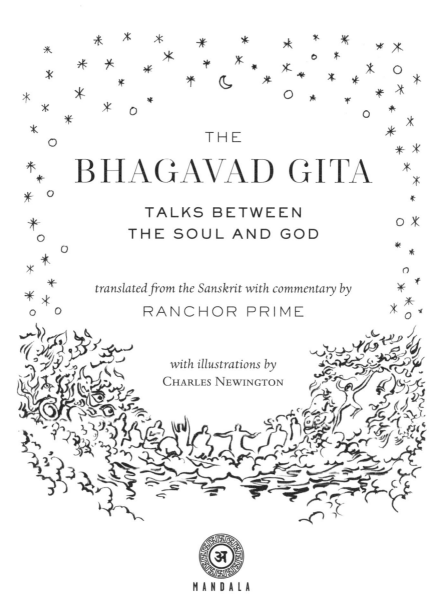

MANDALA

SAN RAFAEL LOS ANGELES LONDON

CONTENTS

| | Preface | ix |
| | Introduction | xi |

PART ONE   THE SOUL IN THE WORLD

ONE	Arjuna's Dilemma	3
TWO	Understanding the Soul	11
THREE	Karma Yoga: Work and Desire	29
FOUR	Transcendental Wisdom	41
FIVE	Life of Freedom	52
SIX	Mystic Yoga	60

PART TWO   THE MYSTERY OF GOD

SEVEN	God and His Energies	75
EIGHT	Attaining the Supreme	83
NINE	Most Confidential Knowledge	92
TEN	God's Infinity	104
ELEVEN	Vision of the Universal Form	114
TWELVE	The Way of Devotion	126

PART THREE   THE JOURNEY

THIRTEEN	Nature and the Soul	137
FOURTEEN	The Three Qualities of Nature	146
FIFTEEN	The Supreme Person	155
SIXTEEN	Light and Dark	163
SEVENTEEN	Three Kinds of Faith	172
EIGHTEEN	The Final Message	180

	Topics in the Bhagavad Gita	200
	Glossary	202
	Index	205

PREFACE

The Gita is a living voice of love and wisdom that belongs to the whole world. In the heart of the reader who is open to hear, this voice takes birth anew. During the eighteen years since this version first appeared, our world has entered deepening crisis and confusion. In these times we can feel the words of the warrior as he places himself before Krishna: Lord I am confused and overwhelmed—tell me what is best for me.

Each one of us has the capacity to look within and find the inner voice, to meet the divine Friend who lives inside and never leaves. These difficult times are here to bring us to this place where we can experience the light of wisdom and the embrace of the love we all long for. Armed with this inner strength and vision we will discover how we are to act in today's troubled world. The words of Krishna preserved in the Bhagavad Gita guide us to this sacred encounter.

I am grateful to Mandala for carrying this message to a new generation of bright eyes and ears. And I am grateful to you, my reader, for stepping with me on this journey of discovery.

RANCHOR DAS
servant of the servant of the one who plays the flute

1 April 2021

INTRODUCTION

'O Krishna, tell me again of your mystic opulences,
for I never tire of hearing your sweet words.'
Bhagavad Gita, 10.18

Krishna's words in the Bhagavad Gita are the finest introduction to the spiritual tradition of India. Yet like the sun which rises in the East and shines everywhere, they belong to the whole world. When I first heard Krishna's voice, it reached me as an echo from a distant land, from a civilization that remembered truths lost in our divided and confused age. I had been brought up to revere the voice of God in the Bible, and until then I had not heard about Krishna's words in the Gita. Here was the same unmistakable voice of the universal God; I indeed felt the book fulfilled its name: *Bhagavad Gita* means 'Song of God.'

The *Gita* is special among Eastern spiritual teachings because it shows how the experience of God can be found in the ordinary actions of everyday life. This sense of the mystical presence was often supposed to be only for those who foresook the world for a life of prayer and meditation, who lived apart from the rest of us in privileged seclusion. The *Gita*, however, offers this experience to us all, encouraging us to remain in the world and to find God in the practice of our daily work. Such awareness calls us to live in the sanctity of every moment and brings with it the possibility of finding great spiritual joy.

The *Gita* is arranged as a conversation between the soul and God, who appear to us as Arjuna and Krishna. In life they were friends, and the *Gita* makes great play of this: spiritual understanding is found through friendship and trust, and ultimately through love. The dialogue of these two friends invites exploration and deep reflection; it is always ready to tell us more, even after many readings. One of the *Gita*'s best-known proponents of the twentieth century was Mahatma Gandhi. He wrote, 'When doubts haunt me and I see not one ray of hope on the horizon, I turn to the *Gita* and find a verse to comfort me.'

How old is the *Gita*? For the spiritual seeker it matters little, for its knowledge is born of eternity, and it is as alive today as it was when it was first spoken. Most modern scholars suppose it achieved its present Sanskrit form around 500 BC, but the Vedic tradition tells us it is much older, and that Krishna originally spoke the *Gita* five thousand years ago.

The *Gita* occupies a unique place as the one universally accessible text acknowledged by all Hindus. Krishna's message of love, based upon the teachings of the world's earliest body of philosophical writings, the *Vedas* and *Upanishads*, draws together the sublime philosophy of the *Upanishads* with the practical path of yoga. It unites the outer world, in which the soul is immersed in the inconceivable energies of God, with the inner world where the soul sits side by side with the divine person. So the *Gita* brings us to the ultimate conclusion of surrender to a loving God.

By the middle of the first millennium AD, the *Gita* was adopted by Hindu teachers as their standard popular text. In around 800 AD it was singled out by the great Shankara for his famous commentary. All the principal Hindu teachers later commented on it, each according to their particular viewpoint. It was first translated into English by Charles Wilkins in 1785, and has since been published in numerous English editions. Henry David Thoreau wrote in 1854 of the 'stupendous and cosmogonal philosophy of the *Bhagavad Gita*.' Thomas Merton in the 1960s saw the *Gita* 'like the Gospels, teaching us to live in awareness of an inner truth. In obedience to that inner truth we are at last free.' Aldous Huxley described the *Gita* as 'one of the clearest and most comprehensive summaries of the Perennial Philosophy ever to have been made. Hence its enduring value, not only for Indians, but for all mankind.'

Spirit of humility

The speaker of the *Bhagavad Gita* is Krishna, who reveals himself to be the supreme godhead. Krishna is the central figure in the vast *Mahabharata*, the epic history of ancient India, of which the

Gita is but one episode. Krishna's teaching opens on the brink of a cataclysmic battle, the events of which are recounted in the *Mahabharata*. Krishna is asked by his personal friend, the warrior Arjuna, to drive his chariot into the space between the two opposing armies. Once he finds himself in the midst of both armies Arjuna despairs and lays down his arms. He turns to Krishna for spiritual help.

Arjuna's despair is due to the awful prospect of having to kill his own friends and family members, who stand in the opposing army. It is said that Arjuna is an enlightened soul placed in illusion by Krishna, and his experience thus parallels our own: God allows us to fall into the illusion of material life, so that we can better learn who we really are and who we wish to be. The physical site where the *Gita* was spoken is Kurukshetra, eighty miles north of Delhi; but the spiritual place where it can be heard, that inner space of emptiness and doubt, is one we all know.

We all have our battles to fight, brought on by illusion. The most difficult battle is the one we wage daily with our own mind and senses. But even in the midst of adversity we must find the time to pause, as Arjuna did between the opposing armies, to contemplate the mysteries of life and what it is we really seek, opening ourselves to hear the voice of the spirit. In order to do this, to make this radical shift in awareness, we need help. When reading the *Gita* we should remember that it is spoken in such a rare moment to one who has put aside certainty and pride. The spirit of humility that allows us to ask for help is easier to speak of than to practice; yet to learn spiritual truths it is essential to open the heart.

Introduction

DIALOGUE OF THE SPIRIT

Having asked for help, Arjuna enters a dialogue of the spirit. He places his earnest questions, and Krishna patiently answers them. One way that this dialogue arises in the life of the spiritual seeker is through learning from a teacher. Since ancient times aspirants began their search by finding a guru. Whether one is fortunate enough to find a guru or not, the dialogue of the spirit ultimately takes place on the inner plane. All of life is a conversation in which God and the individual soul respond to each other. God responds to our desires, allowing us to discover more of God and God's energies.. In this process of discovering God, I discover myself. The connection between the soul and God is a gift, and this is the heart of Krishna's teaching. Once this is understood, all actions become expressions of this inner link with God.

THE SHAPE OF THE *GITA*

The first six chapters begin with an analysis of the self, which establishes each of us as an eternal being, reincarnated from one body to another in the search for liberation from the cycle of birth and death. Then comes the art of yoga: how to live and act in a way that leads to liberation and to union with God.

Krishna teaches three paths of yoga. Karma yoga, the path of action, means to work without attachment to the results of one's work. *Jnana* (pronounced *gyana*) yoga is the path of knowledge of the spirit through study and contemplation. *Bhakti* yoga is the path of devotion to God. Krishna says that all three of these paths lead to the same goal, yet he concludes by recommending the path of *bhakti* yoga.

The middle six chapters describe the transcendent Supreme Being. They contain the heart of the *Gita*: four seed verses in chapter ten, verses 8–11, which describe Krishna as the source of all, and the divine life shared by the wise who are devoted to Krishna. This life transforms every act into a sacred offering of devotion leading to Krishna. Chapter eleven—one of the greatest mystical passages in world literature—contains the famous vision of the Universal Form. This central section of the *Gita* concludes with devotion to Krishna, described in poetic detail in chapter twelve.

The final six chapters further elaborate these themes, adding a detailed explanation of the three material qualities of goodness, passion and darkness, showing how these qualities manifest in daily life. They include, in chapter sixteen, an intense and cautionary account of the effects of the quality of darkness. The last chapter concludes, from verse 55 onward, with a glorious affirmation of Krishna's love, and his final assurance to the traveler on the path: 'Abandon all kinds of religion and surrender to me alone. I will free you from all sinful reactions. Do not fear.'

WHO IS THIS BOOK FOR?

This edition of the *Bhagavad Gita* is for anyone exploring the spiritual path, of whatever faith or persuasion. I have made a completely fresh translation from the Sanskrit, aiming at simplicity and clarity, and I have added the short commentary of a seeker of truth in the modern world. The *Gita* is extremely condensed: each Sanskrit verse is a pithy statement that builds upon the last, developing complex and interwoven ideas into a closely argued philosophical framework. It utilizes standard Vedic concepts such as karma and yoga that could be studied at length. Inevitably, in translating into simple English, I have simplified the nuances of the original Sanskrit text; but I have not dispensed with the verse format, so that each verse can stand alone as a focus for the reader's contemplation.

I learned the *Gita* from my teacher, Srila A.C. Bhaktivedanta Swami Prabhupada. His name, Bhaktivedanta, means devotion combined with spiritual knowledge. His definitive commentary and translation entitled *Bhagavad Gita As It Is* perfectly combines these qualities. He encouraged his followers to write their own devotional commentaries on the *Gita*. I therefore began this book as a way of giving the great teaching to my own children, and in response to requests for a simple retelling of the *Gita* that would be universal in its appeal.

Many who read the *Gita* for the first time will hear Krishna's words as the voice of God or the inner wisdom of the soul. Some will feel faith in Krishna as the incarnation of God who lived in Northern India five thousand years ago, as a cowherd boy who later became a prince of the Yadu dynasty.

Whether you approach the *Gita* as a seeker after truth, whose mind is open to hear a new voice, or as a faithful devotee seeking Krishna's grace, this edition is intended for you, for in this dialogue of the spirit Krishna lets the choice rest with each one of us:

> *'I have told you this most secret of all secret knowledge.*
> *Reflect over this fully, then do as you wish.'*
>
> *Bhagavad Gita, 18.63*

Acknowledgements

A few words of appreciation for some of the many friends and well-wishers who encouraged this book on its way.

When as a young father I sat down to teach the Gita to my children I had to find a language they could understand. I have long believed that if you can't say something sensibly to a thoughtful child, it's probably not worth saying. Hence my children, with their endless questions, were my teachers. The essential mover in all my writing efforts is my eternal teacher, Srila Prabhupada, who long ago asked me to tell people about Krishna. My friend Ian Roberts assured me that I could and should write this book; Martin Palmer added his abundant encouragement; my spiritual elder brother Jayadvaita Swami freely gave his editorial advice and support. My agent Susan Mears backed me and my publisher Debbie Thorpe gave her timely patronage for the original edition of this book.

For the revised edition, my friend in need Rama Nrsimha lent his support, facilitated by my missionary brother, Mahavishnu Swami, who donated generous sponsorship. Pratima Patel gave her time and dedication. Charles Newington answered my last-minute call to work against the clock and manifest an outstanding set of drawings to illuminate this volume, and finally Miles J Krishnadas proof-read and indexed.

My special thanks will always belong to Lena, my patient companion.

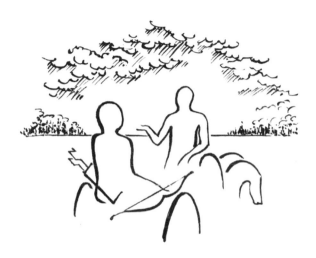

PART ONE

THE SOUL
IN THE WORLD

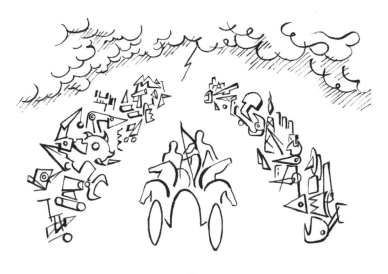

I

Arjuna's Dilemma

The armies prepare to face each other in a battle
that will engulf the known world. The warrior, in
a chariot driven by Krishna, is filled with
foreboding and doubt.

PROLOGUE

The blind monarch Dhritarashtra, whose sons led by Duryodhana will do battle with their cousins the Pandavas, enquires from his trusted secretary:

1

O Sanjaya, what happened once my sons and the sons of Pandu had assembled at the holy field of Kurukshetra, ready to fight?

2

Sanjaya replied:

Once Prince Duryodhana had seen the Pandava armies arrayed against him in battle formation, he spoke to his teacher.

KRISHNA'S TALKS WITH ARJUNA in the *Bhagavad Gita* come to us through the mouth of Sanjaya, gifted with the psychic ability to see and hear faraway events—in this case a distant battlefield. It is clear from the start that this dialogue has a mystical origin.

A more dramatic setting for spiritual teaching could hardly be imagined. The battle which is about to begin will last eighteen days and develop into the most awesome contest of fighting men recorded in ancient history. Yet paradoxically they have chosen a sacred place, the field of Kurukshetra, for this mass slaughter. Reconciling the apparent contradiction between the sacred and the profane is a fundamental concern of the *Bhagavad Gita*.

King Dhritarashtra wants to know what will become of his sons. In response, Sanjaya reports the words of Duryodhana, his chief son, who is addressing his teacher, Dronacharya.

The Field of Battle

3

Duryodhana said:

My teacher, look upon the armies of the Pandavas, commanded by your wise disciple Dhristadyumna.

4-6

There are many heroic warriors equal to their leaders Arjuna and Bhima, such as Yuyudhana, Virata, Drupada, Drstaketu, Chekitana, Kashiraja, Purujit, Kuntibhoja, Shaibya, Yudhamanyu, Uttamauja the son of Subhadra and the sons of Draupadi. All of them are powerful chariot fighters.

7-9

But hear of our own generals, highly qualified to lead our army. There is yourself, Bhishma, Karna, Kripa, Ashvatthama, Vikarna, and Bhurishrava, son of Somadatta. You are all sure to be victorious. Beside you are many other heroes ready to die for my cause. They are all powerfully armed and highly experienced military men.

10-11

Our strength, under the protection of Grandfather Bhishma, cannot be measured; whereas the Pandava's strength, under Bhima, is limited. All of you must now support Bhishma, standing at your appointed places ready for battle.

—*With these words Duryodhana fell silent.*

12–13

The mighty Bhishma, grandfather of the fighters on both sides, sounded his battle conch like the roar of a lion and glad-

dened Duryodhana's heart. The Kuru army vibrated their conches, war drums and horns, making a tumultuous sound.
14-15
Krishna and Arjuna were in a great chariot drawn by four white horses. They sounded their divine conches named Panchajanya and Devadatta. Bhima blew his great conch Paundra.
16-18
Prince Yudhisthira and his fighting companions—among them Nakula, Sahadeva, the King of Varanasi, Shikhandi, Dhristadyumna, Virata, Satyaki, Drupada, the sons of Draupadi and the son of Subhadra—all blew their conches.
19
This combined vibration filled the earth and sky, and shattered the hearts of their opponents.
20
Arjuna stood in his chariot, his bow held at the ready. After scanning the army of the sons of Dhritarashtra, he turned to Krishna.

THE SONS OF DHRITARASHTRA and their cousins, the sons of Pandu, both lay claim to the throne. After years of enmity the two sets of brothers have at last come to settle their differences on the battlefield. They are joined on either side by the military powers of the known world, many of whom are related to one or both parties, all gathered in one place ready to fight to the point of death.

Such is the fate of the powerful: they crush their rivals to gain power, then they in turn are crushed to make room for others. Only Krishna is not part of this remorseless struggle.

He is neutral: he wants nothing, yet he loves all.

War, like a forest fire that cannot be stopped, arises in every generation, causing ordinary people to kill their friends and brothers. It is no accident that such a desperate and confusing time should be chosen by Krishna for delivering his teaching on how to bring an end to suffering.

SURVEYING THE ARMIES

21–23
Arjuna said:
Infallible One, take my chariot between the armies so that I can see who has come here to defend the evil-minded Duryodhana, and with whom I will have to fight.

24–25
Sanjaya narrated:
Obedient to Arjuna's request, Krishna brought the mighty chariot into the middle of the two armies, halting in front of Bhishma, Drona and the chieftains of the world.

Krishna said:
Just behold, Arjuna, all the Kurus assembled here.

26–27
Before him on both sides Arjuna recognized fathers, grandfathers, uncles, brothers, sons, grandsons, teachers and friends. When he saw all these familiar faces confronting one another he was filled with deep compassion and sadness.

ARJUNA HAD NOT WANTED THIS WAR. So it is with each of us: we may not seek conflict, but in response to the choices we make it finds us. Arjuna has made his choices, and Krishna has become

Arjuna's chariot driver to lead him wherever he wishes to go. God does not interfere with our choices. God helps us fulfil them, accompanying each of us as impartial observer of all we do, honoring our freedom. Should our choices lead us into difficulty, God is there as our unseen friend to protect us if we fall.

THE PROSPECT OF DISASTER

28

Arjuna said:

Dear Krishna, when I see these kinsmen in front of me, ready to fight, my limbs weaken and my mouth is parched.

29

My body shivers, my hairs stand on end, my bow slips from my grasp and my skin burns.

30

I can hardly stand. My mind is reeling. I foresee only disaster.

31

No good can come from killing our families. I want no such victory, Krishna, nor the happiness or rewards it might bring.

32–34

What value have power, happiness or life itself, when the ones with whom I would share them—teachers, grandfathers, fathers, sons, grandsons, uncles and brothers—are here to lose everything and die?

35

They may wish to slay me, but I will not kill them even for the whole world.

36

Guilt will haunt us if we kill them. Though Dhritarashtra
and his supporters are aggressors, they do not deserve death.
What happiness could we find by killing our own brothers?

37–38

Blinded by greed, these men see no wrong in killing their
family or friends, yet surely we have the wisdom to shun
such sinful acts.

39

When families are broken, traditions and duties disappear,
and as a result immorality spreads.

40

With the spread of immorality, the chastity of women is lost,
causing the social order to disintegrate.

41

Such disintegration makes hell for everyone—its victims
and its perpetrators. Even the departed souls, deprived of
the prayers and offerings of their families, fall from peace.

42

So the breakdown of the family makes the very foundations
of community fall apart.

43

Moreover, Krishna, I have heard it said that those whose
family traditions are destroyed are destined to live in hell.

44

How terrible that our greed for earthly power should
drive us to such sinful deeds as the destruction of our own
families.

45

It would be better if the sons of Dhritarashtra came with
their weapons and killed me, unarmed and unresisting.

46

Sanjaya concluded:
Speaking so, in the midst of that battlefield, Arjuna dropped his weapons and sank into his chariot, overwhelmed with grief.

THIS OPENING CHAPTER IS SET in an ancient society, yet the issues of morality and social order that concerned Arjuna still concern us today. Justice and defense of the oppressed are obligations for us all, especially in times of conflict when ordinary safeguards break down. Some believe justice requires the application of violence, whereas others, seeing that one person's aggressor is another's father, brother or son, believe forgiveness is the better way. These are the moral dilemmas that have beset humanity since the first humans lived together.

Added to these is the unprecedented dilemma of our times, when humanity is at war with the natural world. In the wisdom tradition of the *Gita* the world is our own Mother. This conflict threatens to destroy us all, and calls us to a profound reassessment of our relationship with all of life.

Faced with the prospect of disaster, Arjuna's heart says one thing and his head another. Confusion and emotion battle in his warrior's chest. This is the context for the *Bhagavad Gita*. The calm voice of truth must enter like clear sunlight on a darkened road. The stage is set for Krishna to teach Arjuna, and through him all those troubled or inquisitive souls who would listen to his words of wisdom.

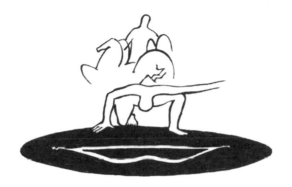

2

UNDERSTANDING THE SOUL

After laying down his bow and refusing to fight
the warrior implores Krishna's help.
Krishna teaches that the soul is eternal and yoga
is the soul's path to freedom.

ARJUNA'S SORROW

1

Arjuna was overcome with compassion and sorrow. His eyes filled with tears. Seeing this, Krishna began to speak.

2

The Blessed Lord said:

Dear Arjuna, how has this despondency come over you in the hour of crisis? This is not the way of a noble person like you. It will lead you not to heaven, but to disgrace.

3

Do not give in to this frailty. It does not become you. Abandon this weakness of heart and prepare to fight.

4

Arjuna replied:

O Krishna, how can I aim my arrows at men like Bhishma and Drona, who are worthy of my worship?

5

I would rather become a beggar than kill these great souls who are my teachers. If for the sake of worldly gain I kill my superiors, my victory will be stained with their blood.

6

I do not know which is better: to conquer them or to be conquered by them. If I were to kill the sons of Dhritarashtra who stand before me, I would have no more reason to live.

TEARS MARK ARJUNA AS OPEN TO HEAR spiritual truths. In times of crisis, when the uncertainties and pain of this world bear down, we may at last be ready to part the veil of material illusion and hear the truth. However, though tears may be a sign of compassion, they are also a sign of illusion. We long to relieve the suffering of the body and mind, but we do not know how.

The body and mind are only the outer dress of the eternal self. If we wish to end suffering, we must care not just for the body and mind, but also for the inner eternal self. This eternal self will be the main subject for Krishna's first discourse.

We are reminded here that the speaker, Krishna, is named *Bhagavan*, which means 'Possessor of Opulence.' During his life on earth he radiated the six opulences of beauty, wisdom, strength, wealth, fame and detachment. For those ready to hear, his words will resound with these qualities to drive away illusion and its companion, suffering.

SUBMISSION BEFORE KRISHNA

7

I am confused about my duty and overwhelmed with weakness. I surrender to you as your disciple and beg you to teach me what is best for me.

8

Nothing will drive away this burning sorrow, even if I win an unrivalled kingdom on earth with the powers of a god.

9

Krishna, I shall not fight.

—*With these words the great warrior fell silent.*

10

Between the two armies Krishna smiled and spoke to the sorrowful Arjuna.

ARJUNA IS NOW READY to accept Krishna as his spiritual teacher. When we are overwhelmed by life's complexities we do well to accept help with openness and humility. To learn from a teacher one must abandon pride and ask for guidance. This is the right spirit with which to hear Krishna's words in the Bhagavad Gita.

Krishna smiles because he is confident he will soon dispel his friend's misery, but he does not comfort Arjuna. Instead, Krishna's words will be uncompromising and direct, because his purpose is to teach the truth.

THE SELF IS DIFFERENT FROM THE BODY

11

The Blessed Lord said:

You speak learned words, but you mourn for what is not worth your sorrow. The wise do not lament for the living or the dead.

12

There was never a time when I did not exist, nor you, nor all these warriors. Nor will there be a time when any of us shall not exist.

13

As the one within this body moves from childhood to youth to old age, so it passes into another body at death. The wise are not confused by this change.

HERE IS THE ESSENTIAL UNDERSTANDING of reincarnation. The self inside the body is eternal. One who knows this has no need to lament for the body, which is a temporary covering for the self.

Krishna describes all those present as eternal beings who pass from one temporary body to another. Each of us can experience this process of change for ourselves. We see our childhood body change to that of an adult, and our adult body to that of an old person. Medical science tells us that the cells in our bodies are constantly being replaced. Despite these outer changes we still feel ourselves inwardly to be the same person: the essence of the inner self does not change. According to this teaching, when at last the outer body dies this inner self moves on to enter a new body.

TOLERATE THE IMPERMANENT

14

Happiness and distress appear and disappear like winter and summer. They arise from the perceptions of the senses and you must learn to tolerate them without being disturbed.

15

When one is undisturbed by happiness and distress and is steady in both, one is fit for eternal life.

16

The unreal has no permanent existence; the real exists forever without change. So conclude seers of the truth who have studied the nature of both.

WE ARE ETERNAL BEINGS, YET WE EXPERIENCE through our senses and mind the ever-changing conditions of this temporary world, from the cold of winter to the heat of summer. If we practice patience in the face of the pleasures and pains of life and the happiness and distress they bring, we will learn to distinguish the firm ground of truth, which is eternal, from the tides of illusion.

ETERNAL SELF

17

That which pervades the body is indestructible. No one can destroy this imperishable one.

18

The body in which this eternal, indestructible and immeasurable one lives must come to an end. Therefore fight, Arjuna.

19

Some think this one is slayer, some think it is slain. Both are wrong, for it is neither slayer nor slain.

20

It exists forever in the present, having no birth or death. It is the oldest, without beginning or end, and is not killed when the body is killed.

21

When one knows this to be indestructible, eternal, without birth or change, how can one possibly kill or induce anyone else to kill?

22

As a person exchanges old clothes for new, so the self abandons old bodies to enter new ones.

23

This self cannot be cut by weapons, burned by fire, drenched by water or withered by wind.

24

It cannot be pierced, burned, wet or dried. For it is ever-lasting, all pervading, unchangeable and immovable, staying eternally the same.

25

It is said that this unchanging one is invisible and inconceivable. Knowing this, you should not lament.

BY NATURE'S LAW, WHATEVER IS BORN MUST DIE. But the self has no birth and hence no death: the soul is life itself. We can perceive the presence of the sun by its warmth and light, even when it is hidden behind clouds. In the same way we can perceive the presence of the self by the life it gives to the body. This life we call consciousness, and it is indestructible.

Here is further explanation of the process of reincarnation, through which the self takes on new identities, as an actor changes dress to play new parts. This change of body is made possible by the grace of God, who fulfils our desires as one friend fulfils the desires of another. We are never separated from God, who accompanies each one of us from one body to the next on our journey through the universe. Though we are forgetful, God knows our past, present and future, and Krishna's words in the *Bhagavad Gita* awaken us to who we really are.

Each individual being is a part of the Supreme Soul, a spark of the divine fire. As a spark possesses the qualities of the fire in minute proportion, so each conscious being possesses in minute quantity the qualities of the Supreme Soul. As the Supreme Soul is indestructible, so is each particle. Each one has a unique identity, never to be lost or dissolved. To awaken our eternal identity as a companion of God is the greatest goal of life.

Do Not Lament

26

O mighty-armed Arjuna, even if you believe this one is forever born and forever dying, still you should not lament.

27

One who is born must die, and one who dies must be reborn. Do not mourn the inevitable.

28

All beings are invisible in the beginning, visible in the middle, and invisible in the end. Why grieve over this?

29

Some have direct experience of this, whereas some only hear or speak about it. All these find it wonderful. Others, though they hear about it, cannot understand it at all.

30

The one who lives in the body can never be killed. Therefore you should not lament for any living being.

THE SOUL IS A THING OF WONDER, yet most of us are too preoccupied with the external world to contemplate it. Without knowing who or what we are we struggle for existence, unaware that the solution to all our problems is found in self-under-standing.

Krishna's words, spoken on a battlefield, leave no room for sentimentality. Everything in this world must disappear in the end. However, taking the life of another creature, even though the self lives on unharmed, interferes with that being's destiny. Killing brings its reaction for the perpetrator.

THE HONORABLE WARRIOR

31

Do not hesitate in your sacred duty as a warrior. For a soldier nothing is more sacred than the fight for a just cause.

32

Fortunate is the warrior for whom this opportunity comes, opening the doors of heaven.

33

If you do not take up this just fight, you will fail in your duty and your honor will be lost.

34

People will forever speak of your shame, and for one who has been honored, dishonor is worse than death.

35–36

The great warriors who gave you honor will think you have fled the battlefield. They will scorn you and your enemies will deride you. What could be more painful?

37

If you die in battle you will enter heaven. If you win you will enjoy the earth. Therefore rise and fight with determination.

38

Fight for the sake of fighting. Look equally on happiness or distress, gain or loss, victory or defeat. In this way you will not incur sin.

THE DUTY OF THE STRONG IS TO PROTECT the weak. The scriptures promise birth in heavenly realms to a warrior who dies fighting for such a just cause. There are many levels of existence within the material world. The heavenly realms lie above the earthly plane, but they are still within the world of birth and death.

Krishna here completes his teaching about the soul. He will now teach how the soul should act to get free from the binding ropes of karma.

In this world of birth and death we are all called to fight in the daily struggle of life, where every action produces a reaction that binds us to the cycle of rebirth. The literal meaning of the Sanskrit word karma is 'action' or 'work.' It also refers to the reactions of work that bind the soul. Karma yoga is the art of work with no reaction.

PATH OF FREEDOM

39

Now I have taught you in detail about the self. Next, hear about yoga, or work without attachment. When you act with this knowledge you can free yourself from the bondage of action.

40

On this path there can be no loss or disappointment. Even a little progress on this path will free you from great fear.

41

Those on this path are resolute and single-minded. The thoughts of those who lack such determination branch endlessly in all directions.

HUMAN LIFE OFFERS FREEDOM from the cycle of birth and death through spiritual development. Even a little progress along the path of spiritual development lasts forever, while material development brings only temporary benefits. At the very least, spiritual activities guarantee a human birth in the next life, from which further spiritual progress can be made. Thus we are saved from passing into a non-human body in the next life, where we will have no opportunity for self-understanding.

When our activities are connected to Krishna through awareness of him as the goal, our lives achieve a unity of purpose that is deeply satisfying. Without such unity of purpose the mind will be full of endless desires and we will never be at peace.

BEYOND THE REWARDS OF PARADISE

42–43

Those without knowledge are drawn only to the ritual and poetry of the scriptures and the rewards they promise, such as birth in paradise. They long for pleasure and power and care for little else.

44

Carried away by their love of pleasure and power, they lack the inner resolve for spiritual life.

45

The rituals of religion belong to this world. Rise above them, Arjuna, above the dualities of pleasure and pain and ambition for profit and security. Be fixed in truth and centered in your inner self.

46

For one who knows the ocean of truth, these rituals are no more than a small pond in the midst of a vast flood.

THE SCRIPTURES OF THE WORLD promise rewards in paradise, but none of these will last forever. Those attached to pleasure and power will have to remain in the world of birth and death, even after enjoying paradise.

For those willing to discover their true spiritual selves, the *Vedas* include the *Upanishads* and the *Bhagavad Gita*. These sacred texts lead from the world of the temporary to the world of the eternal. The goal of all scriptures is to remember God. A life overflooded by remembrance of Krishna's name has no need for the rituals of religion or the rewards they bring. These rituals appear as a small pond in the presence of the ocean.

THE ART OF ALL WORK

47

You have the right to work, but not to its results. Do not be attached to the fruits of work, or to not working.

48

Work with a spirit of detachment, being equal to success or failure. Such evenness of mind is called yoga.

49

Through the practice of yoga, avoid selfish work and surrender yourself to the guidance of inner divine wisdom. Those who seek rewards from work do not find happiness.

50

One who is guided by divine wisdom passes beyond good
and bad actions. Therefore strive for yoga, the art of all work.

THE RESULTS OF ACTIONS ARE CALLED by Krishna the fruits of
work. Every action produces a fruit: some sweet, some bitter.
Those who want to enjoy the fruits of their work are bound to
the cycle of birth and death to fulfil their desires. Even good
deeds, if done with attachment, draw us back to this world to
taste their results. This attachment can be overcome by working
for the sake of Krishna. Yoga means living in awareness of God.

As we will learn in later chapters, Krishna is the root of all
existence. When the root of the cosmic tree is watered, the
leaves and branches are nourished. By working for Krishna we
benefit ourselves and the whole world. This is the key to happiness and the end to suffering. This kind of work in loving service
brings the guidance of inner wisdom, called here *buddhi yoga,* or
direct communion with the Lord in the heart.

LEAVING THE FOREST

51

The wise, guided by divine wisdom, free themselves from
the cycle of birth and death by letting go of the results of
their actions. So they reach the place beyond all miseries.

52

When your intelligence has passed out of the forest of delusion you will become indifferent to all that has been heard
and all that is to be heard.

53

Your mind will be secure in self-knowledge and undisturbed by the voices of wordly religion and ritual. Then you will have achieved true yoga.

THE SENSE OF PERSONAL OWNERSHIP IN THIS WORLD and the attachment it brings are an illusion, for all belongs to God. Those who understand this leave aside attachment for earthly rewards and are released from the world of birth and death. Many have trod this path of detachment, inspired by love for God, and their example and words go before us.

THE UNDISTURBED ONE

54
Arjuna asked:

How will I recognize one who has understood the self? How would such an enlightened one sit, or move or speak?

55
Krishna said:

One who does not dwell on the desires in the mind, but finds satisfaction within, is deep in knowledge.

56

One who is undisturbed by misery, not craving happiness, free from attachment, fear and anger, is a sage of steady mind.

57

One who is without affection for good or evil, meeting both without praise or blame, is secure in wisdom.

INNER CONCENTRATION AND STILLNESS, called *samadhi*, is the first symptom of the enlightened soul. This state of mind overcomes the craving for material pleasure that is the cause of so much unhappiness. In the world of matter, in which the senses predominate, the mind gravitates toward sense enjoyment. However, if one finds spiritual happiness within, one finds a contentment more satisfying than anything sense enjoyment can offer. In this position the natural good qualities of the soul develop of their own accord. A person who lives in this way is freed from attachment, fear and anger and accepts the good and bad of this world equally as the mercy of God.

THE POWER OF THE SENSES

58

One who withdraws the senses from the world, as a tortoise draws in its limbs, is secure in wisdom.

59

You may renounce external pleasures but still desire to enjoy them. Such desires cease only when you taste a higher reality.

60

The senses are so strong that they can carry away the mind even of a wise person striving to subdue them.

61

One who restrains the senses and whose thoughts are focused on me is secure in wisdom.

62

While dwelling on the objects of the senses, you develop attachment for them. From attachment grows desire and from desire arises anger.

63

Anger produces illusion, and from illusion comes forget-fulness. Forgetfulness destroys your intelligence, and when intelligence is gone you are lost.

THE SENSES MAKE GOOD SERVANTS but bad masters. It is natural to enjoy the senses, yet sense enjoyment brings suffering in its wake. This is the puzzle of material existence. On the spiritual path one must bring the senses under control, as a sick person must follow a restricted diet to get healthy. However, unless one tastes the inner satisfaction of the soul, artificial restrictions lead to frustration and the taste for material pleasure persists.

FREEDOM IN SELF-CONTROL

64

One who practices self-control, who engages with the world without attraction or aversion, achieves the mercy of God.

65

This mercy ends all miseries. In this serene state the intelligence soon becomes clear.

66

One without self-control cannot have a clear intelligence or a steady mind. An unsteady mind finds no peace, and without peace where is joy?

67

As a strong wind sweeps away a boat on the water, so the mind dwelling on even one of the senses carries away the intelligence.

68

Therefore one whose senses are under control is secure in wisdom.

THE SELF-CONTROL OF YOGA BRINGS FREEDOM from attraction and aversion, the opposing forces that govern material life. One must sacrifice the apparent freedom of sense gratification to gain the real freedom of inner peace that comes by the grace of God.

In the yoga of devotion the senses are controlled not by force, but by attraction to the higher principle of loving service to Krishna. The eyes of devotion see that everyone in this world is dear to Krishna, and Krishna is the dearest friend of everyone. This simple truth provides a calm center for the mind, and so lasting peace and happiness.

PEACE IN THE NIGHT

69

Night in this world is the time of awakening for the self-controlled, and the time of awakening in this world is night for those with inner vision.

70

One who is undisturbed by the flow of desires finds peace, as the ocean, though filled by incessant rivers, remains still. One who strives to satisfy those desires finds no peace.

71

One who gives up selfish desires, who lives content, without ego or possessiveness, achieves peace.

72

This is the spiritual path, on which you will not be deluded.
If you follow this path, even at the hour of death, you will
enter the presence of God.

LASTING PEACE IS FOUND IN THE PRESENCE of God. God is present everywhere and we are always in God's presence. The flow of desires and our attachment to them obscure our perception of this divine presence. The essence of Krishna's advice in this second chapter is to abandon selfish desires. Then it will be possible to perceive the presence and the will of God.

Those unaware of God's will live in illusion, and their day seems like night to the God-aware. Conversely, those who serve the will of God appear from the material point of view to be in illusion: their day also seems like night. So a fundamental divergence exists between the spiritual and the material ways of life.

Service to God satisfies the soul so much that it fills the spiritual aspirant with inner peace, deep and still like the ocean. In this state the flow of material desires, so avidly promoted by the commercial interests of the world, passes unnoticed.

Desires are natural to the soul and cannot be negated. The soul yearns for the presence of God because each soul is an eternal child of God and shares the same spiritual nature. We do not have to wait for death in order to enter the presence of God. We have only to absorb ourselves in his loving service to have already attained the spiritual kingdom. This can take many lifetimes or it can be achieved within a second.

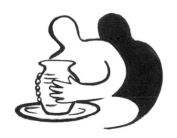

3
KARMA YOGA: WORK AND DESIRE

The wheel of sacrifice brings welfare to all who help it turn. The enemy of this world is selfish desire, destroyer of self understanding.

THE NEED TO ACT

1

Arjuna said:

Krishna, if you think knowledge is superior to action, why urge me to fight this terrible battle?

2

I am confused by your contradictory words. Please tell me clearly which path will lead me to the highest good.

3

The Supreme Person said:

Arjuna, long ago I explained two paths of faith in this world: the contemplative are inclined to the path of knowledge, and the active to the path of service.

4

One cannot gain freedom just by avoiding work, and mere renunciation will not bring success.

5

No one can be still even for a moment, for all are compelled against their will to act according to their natures.

6

One who outwardly controls the senses while inwardly dwelling on sense enjoyment is deluded and is a pretender.

7

But one who inwardly controls the senses while outwardly working without attachment is on the right path.

8

Do the work alotted to you. Action is better than inaction. Without work you cannot even maintain your body.

ACTIVITY IS FUNDAMENTAL TO THE SELF, for the nature of the soul
is to give to others and ultimately to give to the Lord. Therefore we must all work if we are to be happy. Work that seeks to
control others or take from them creates conflict and unhappiness, whereas work in the spirit of service leads the soul toward
satisfaction and knowledge.

Knowledge and action belong side by side in spiritual life,
for philosophy without faith is dry speculation; and faith without philosophy is sentiment, which gives rise to fanaticism.
Philosophy and honest work belong together.

THE WHEEL OF SACRIFICE

9

Do your work as a sacrifice for Vishnu, or it will bind you
to this world. Work for his sake and you will always be free.

10

In the beginning the Creator sent generations of beings into
the world along with sacrifice, saying, 'Be happy and pros-
per, for sacrifice will bring you all that you desire.'

11

The heavenly beings nourished by your sacrifice will also
nourish you. Pleasing one another, you will all achieve the
highest benefit.

12

Satisfied by your offerings, those heavenly beings will give
you all you wish for. But one who enjoys their gifts without
giving in return is a thief.

13

Gentle people, who offer their food before eating, are released from all sins. The unfortunate, who cook only for themselves, eat suffering.

14

Life is sustained by food grains. Food grains are nourished by rains. Rains depend on sacrifice and sacrifice is born of work.

15

Work comes from the Vedas and the Vedas arise from the Supreme Godhead. Therefore the all-pervading Transcend-ence is eternally situated in acts of sacrifice.

16

So turns the wheel of sacrifice. One who lives selfishly, who delights only in the senses and does not care for the turning of this wheel, lives in vain.

GIFTS SUCH AS RAIN AND FOOD depend on the great cycle outlined here by Krishna. All work forms part of this cycle, called here the wheel of sacrifice. This cosmic cycle guarantees us all we need. Our survival depends not on the results of our work, but on the goodwill of the heavenly beings, called *Devas*. Their service to God is to look after our needs, and we in turn must serve them. Life is thus a process of giving and receiving in which we depend upon each other for happiness and security. Those who neglect this cosmic cycle, in Krishna's words, 'live in vain.'

To harmonize our work with this cycle we need Krishna's guidance. The universe teaches how to live in this spirit, and its books of guidance are the *Vedas*, breath of the Lord. The original *Vedas* were in the form of Sanskrit hymns; but their wisdom is encoded in all the scriptures of the world. They, and the saints who follow them, point the way to happiness and spiritual enlightenment. By following their divine wisdom we can deepen our relationship with God, and at the same time fulfil our desires in this world.

The best way to satisfy the *Devas* is to dedicate our work to the Supreme Lord, the root of all existence. For example, prayer, or the simple chanting of God's names, transforms all work into divine service, as does the daily offering of our food to God. Such sanctified food loosens the bonds of karma and purifies our existence. These two practices, prayer and eating sanctified food, are enough to transform our whole existence.

WORK WITH DETACHMENT

17
However, one who finds pleasure within, who is illuminated within, who is satisfied in the self alone—such a person has no need to work.

18
This person has nothing to gain or lose by working or by not working, and does not depend on any being for anything.

19
Thus do your work without attachment, for by working without personal motive you will reach the Supreme.

THE SIGN OF THE ENLIGHTENED STATE of consciousness is that a person finds pleasure within. The nature of the soul is to seek pleasure. Thus, so long as we do not taste that inner peace, called here *atmarati*, 'pleasure in the self,' we will be drawn to the external pleasures of the world and will bind ourselves to the cycle of attachment.

By tasting inner happiness we are freed, and our path becomes clear to work for the sake of the Lord, unattached to personal gain. In this stage our work is revealed to us from within, illuminated by the grace of God.

THE WELFARE OF ALL

20

Janaka and others reached perfection by working in this way. So you, for the welfare of all, should do the same.

21

Whatever a great person does, others imitate. The standards set by the great are followed by all the world.

22

I have no duty, nor is there anything in all the three worlds that I need or want—yet even I work.

23

For if I did not work tirelessly, surely all humans would follow my path.

24

If I were not to work, the worlds would fall into ruin. I would bring chaos and destroy the peace of all beings.

25

As the ignorant act for themselves, so the wise should also act, but selflessly for the benefit of the world.

THE WORK OF MAINTENANCE IS HIDDEN from the maintained, as parents' efforts in running a household are hidden from their children. Thus we cannot understand how Krishna works for our welfare. Yet if we observe the wonders of creation we can see everywhere signs of divine care for all beings. God's work sets the pattern for us all. By working in a spirit of selflessness, for the benefit of others, we can share in the nature of God and be freed from the ties of this world.

DO NOT UNSETTLE THE IGNORANT

26

A wise person does not disturb the minds of the ignorant who are attached to their work, but acts in the spirit of devotion and encourages them to do the same.

27

Material nature does everything. Yet, deluded by ego, the soul thinks, 'I am the doer.'

28

One who knows the truth, Arjuna, sees how nature acts and becomes detached from the senses and their objects.

29

Bewildered by nature's ways, fools are caught up in her works. Yet the wise should not unsettle those whose understanding is incomplete.

SO LONG AS WE REMAIN IN THE ILLUSION of material life, we attach ourselves to the material body and take it for granted that we are doing everything by ourselves. We are unaware that our actions are made possible by the Lord, and that on our own we can do nothing.

Souls in this world are absorbed in their activities like dreamers in their dreams. Each soul has a particular course to pursue, and only when the time is right, when the dream becomes too painful or too plain, will the soul be ready to perceive another reality. Then, as a sleeper awakens when called by name, the soul awakens on hearing the name of Krishna.

CHOOSE TO BE FREE

30
Devote your actions to me and fix your mind on the Self.
Forgetting selfish desires, fight without hesitation.
31
Those who follow this teaching of mine, faithfully and with open hearts, are freed from the bondage of karma.
32
Be assured that those who have no regard for these teachings and do not follow them will be misguided and lost.

WE CANNOT BE HAPPY WITHOUT GOD. The Supreme Lord is the Soul of all souls, on whom our existence depends. Yet our spiritual nature is to be free. The resolution of this paradox is to choose freely the service of God. This means to choose the way of loving and giving, for only that will satisfy the soul. This is what Krishna wishes us to understand by saying, 'Devote your actions to me, fixing your mind on the Self,' for Krishna is the Self of our self.

Faith in the Lord's orders, even if we are not perfect in following them, is enough to bring liberation—this is Krishna's promise. It is a matter of intention and disposition, not performance. Sincerity of purpose is all that is asked, for we each have our own abilities and limitations, as Krishna will explain.

If we choose to disregard the Lord's teachings, as they are found in the *Bhagavad Gita* or other sacred books of the world, God will not interfere with our choice. By so deciding, we choose to remain under the spell of the illusions of the material world until we are ready to choose again.

WALK THE PATH GIVEN TO YOU

33
Even the wise act according to their natures, for all beings follow nature. What can repression accomplish?
34
Attraction and aversion that govern the senses are obstacles on your path—do not let them rule you.
35
The occupation given to you, though imperfect, is better than another's, even perfectly done. Defeat on one's own path is better; for another's path is dangerous.

IT IS BEST TO KNOW OUR LIMITATIONS and work honestly from our natural level, rather than try to be other than we really are. If I accept a path meant for someone else, whether it is more or less demanding than my own, and deny my own nature and disposition, I will be led to disappointment and frustration. Once I find my own occupation and dedicate myself to pursuing it in the service of God or God's creation, I will find fulfilment.

This verse 35 about finding your natural occupation is repeated for emphasis in the eighteenth chapter, verse 47.

The process of spiritual development is a gradual one, not abrupt. If we patiently follow the recommended process, in course of time we will transcend material considerations and be able to attempt anything for the sake of Krishna.

THE ENEMY WITHIN

36
Arjuna said:
Krishna, what drives people to commit sinful acts even unwillingly, as if by force?
37
The Lord said:
It is desire, born of passion and later transformed into wrath, that is the all-devouring sinful enemy of this world.
38
As fire is covered by smoke, as a mirror by dust, as an embryo by the womb, so knowledge is covered by desire.
39
Thus knowledge is veiled by desire, the eternal enemy of the wise, which is never satisfied and burns like fire.
40
It lives in the senses, the mind, and the intelligence, using them to cover knowledge and bewilder the living being.

41

Therefore first control your senses, Arjuna, then slay this
sinful destroyer of knowledge and self-realisation.

42

The senses are elevated; above them is the mind; above the
mind is the intelligence; and even higher than the intelligence is the self.

43

Knowing yourself to be transcendental to the intelligence,
steady your lower self by your higher self and defeat this
formidable enemy called desire.

MATERIAL DESIRE, DESCRIBED HERE as the enemy, is called *kama*
in Sanskrit. The pure form of desire, however, is called *prema*,
'divine love,' the original basis of all emotions. When the soul's
eternal love is directed toward God's creation instead of toward
God it is transmuted into *kama*, or material desire. This *kama*,
when frustrated, produces anger.

So long as we are under the control of material desire we
will have to gratify the demands of the mind and senses. In
return we may feel some happiness; but this happiness is limited
and temporary, and because it leads to frustration is the enemy
of the true self.

Thus in the material world the living entity is bound by
the golden shackles of *kama*, particularly in the form of sexual
desire. No amount of gratification will satisfy *kama*, just as no
amount of fuel added to a fire will extinguish it. When the soul's
search for pleasure in matter is at last baffled, the soul is ready to

discover its true nature. This inquiry is the start of the spiritual path and is the most important quest of human life.

The process of restoring true knowledge begins with understanding the difference between the self and the body, and with meditation upon the Supreme Lord. When the intelligence and mind are thus steadied and restored, we can gradually bring the senses under control. Thus *kama* can be transmuted into love, and the enemy slain.

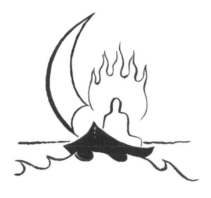

4

TRANSCENDENTAL WISDOM

Krishna descends to earth to re-establish
the knowledge of yoga which burns karma to
ashes. The boat of this knowledge will carry you
over the ocean of misery.

DESCENT OF WISDOM

1

The Blessed Lord said:

I taught this eternal yoga to Vivasvan the sun god; Vivasvan gave it to Manu, father of mankind; Manu passed it to King Iksvaku.

2

Thus handed from one to another, it was known by saintly kings. But over a great passage of time this yoga was lost to the world.

3

Now I am teaching the transcendental secret of this ancient yoga to you, Arjuna, because you are my devotee and my friend.

THE VEDIC CIVILIZATION, LIKE OTHER ancient civilizations, saw its past as a time of wisdom lost to a later age. In modern times, dazzled by the advancement of science and communications, some of us have come to look upon old knowledge as inferior to our own. However, truths do not change, only our perception of them. A new truth to one person may be an old truth to another. Yoga is such a truth.

The Vedic rulers claimed descent from the Sun, and hence they took the name *Suryavamsa*, meaning dynasty of the Sun. They brought the knowledge of yoga to earth during the reign of Iksvaku, by Vedic calculations two million years ago. The sacred duty of the *Suryavamsa* was to safeguard and teach this wisdom, which gave meaning and order to human life. Krishna revived the knowledge of yoga when he taught Arjuna.

Krishna chose to teach yoga to Arjuna because Arjuna was devoted to him. Devotion is the quality that makes a person receptive to spiritual wisdom. Scrutiny and inquiry are necessary in the search for truth, but they come best from a mind and heart that is open. The way to understand Krishna is the same as the way to understand any person—with love.

KRISHNA'S MISSION

4

Arjuna said:

Vivasvan was born long before you. How am I to understand that originally you taught him?

5

The Blessed Lord said:

Arjuna, both you and I have both passed many births. I remember them all, but you do not.

6

I am the Lord of all beings, without birth or death, yet still I appear in this world in my original divine form.

7

Whenever and wherever there is a decline in religion and a rise of materialism, at that time I manifest myself in this world.

8

To protect the good, to subdue the harmful and to reestablish the principles of religion, I appear in every age.

9

One who understands the divine nature of my birth and actions is not reborn after leaving this body, but comes to me, Arjuna.

As THE SUN APPEARS TO RISE AND SET, so the Lord appears to be born and to die. And like the sun, the Lord is seen in many lands and many epochs, for he expands in countless forms while remaining One. When he descends into this world, he speaks the truth in a way that can be heard by the people of that place and time. He appears personally or he sends his son or his servant. Krishna, the Buddha and Jesus are among his divine appearances.

Krishna appears in this world in his eternal spiritual form, which is one and the same with himself. We each share in Krishna's nature, yet we forget ourselves when we enter the cycle of birth and death. Krishna never forgets: he remembers everything, always and everywhere. In his many descents into this world Krishna brings his eternal companions, such as Arjuna, who was with Krishna when he spoke to the sun god millions of years previously. As Krishna accompanies Arjuna through many births, so he accompanies each of us as our silent helper and protector. Without him this world would fall into ruin, and without his silent love and support we would be lost.

FREEDOM FROM FEAR AND ANGER

10

Freed from attachment, fear and anger, with mind absorbed in me and illuminated by me, many sought refuge in me and so gained love for me.

11

As they seek my shelter, so I reveal to them my love. All beings everywhere are on my path.

12

Those in search of worldly success serve the gods of this world. For here on earth the results of work come quickly.

13

According to their natures and work, I divided humans into four classes. Yet though I did this, know that I am changeless and do nothing.

14

Work does not affect me; nor do I seek its rewards. One who knows this truth about me is not bound by work.

15

Long ago, those seeking freedom worked with this understanding. So should you, following their ancient example.

KRISHNA CREATED THE MANY PATHS upon which we all walk. Whatever a person's desires, Krishna allows and facilitates those desires. He is the friend of all.

People desire wealth or fame, and for it they sacrifice to the gods and the powerful of this world. But the rewards they receive are limited and temporary, and attachment to them brings fear and anger. Frustration, repression, fear of failure, fear of knowing oneself—these symptoms arise when we attach ourselves to the temporary forms of the material world and forget our eternal identities.

Therefore Krishna advises us to continue working, but without attachment and with knowledge. For the paths and ways of work created by him are formed so as to encourage us to rediscover our real natures, and again share with love and freedom in Krishna's spiritual existence.

The path to spiritual enlightenment will demand all our determination. Yet Krishna assures us that many have trod this path in the past and been successful. The encouragement of fellow spiritual travelers is essential. Even in this modern age many are walking this path.

HOW KARMA WORKS

16

What is action and what is inaction? This question confuses even the wise. I shall teach you about action, so you can be free from harm.

17

The ways of action are hard to know. You must learn to distinguish action, forbidden action and inaction.

18

One who sees inaction in action, and action in inaction, is truly wise and on the spiritual path, though doing all kinds of work.

19

One whose enterprises are without selfish motive, whose karmic reactions are consumed in the fire of knowledge, the wise call learned.

20

One who renounces the results of work, being content and self-sufficient, though fully occupied in work, does nothing.

21

One who is without motive, with mind and intelligence controlled, with no sense of ownership, though working to sustain life, incurs no sin.

22

One who is satisfied with gain that comes of its own accord, who is above the dualities of this world, free of envy and steady in success and failure, though working, is not bound by karma.

23

For one who relinquishes all attachment, absorbed in knowledge, acting only in sacrifice, all work merges into transcendence.

24

A person absorbed in spiritual work sees the whole process of sacrifice—the giver and the gift, the offering and its acceptance—as pure spirit, and so enters the spiritual nature.

WORK IS DIVINE. To practice this understanding three kinds of work must be distinguished: work to be avoided, work that binds, and work that frees.

Work that should be avoided is defined in Vedic tradition by four moral codes prohibiting meat-eating, gambling, intoxication and promiscuous sex. The principle is that any activity which needlessly harms or exploits another living being, or one's own self, should be avoided. Work that binds is any work done with attachment to the results, and work that frees is any work done without attachment to the results.

The entire cycle of work—the worker, the endeavour, the instruments, the intention and the result—is all *Brahman*, the divine energy of God. Originally all is spirit. Only when spirit is used for selfish ends does it appear to be material. Recognising the spiritual origin of everything transforms our lives—the same work that once caused bondage becomes the cause of liberation. Knowing Krishna is my protector, I can place my welfare in his hands, accept whatever gain comes of its own accord, and work for the welfare of all beings. So I become free.

THE WAYS OF SACRIFICE

25

Some mystics give sacrifices to the heavenly beings, and others give them in the fire of the Supreme Spirit.

26

Some give the senses such as hearing into the fire of self-restraint, and others give the objects of the senses such as sound into the fire of the senses.

27

Some give the work of the senses and of the life force into the yogic fire of the controlled mind to gain knowledge of the self.

28

Others give their possessions, or perform penances, or practice yoga, or study the Vedas while following strict vows.

29

Others, inclined to breath control, give their outward breath to their inward and their inward breath to their outward, stilling both. Or they restrict their diet and offer the outward breath to itself.

30

All these who understand sacrifice are released from their sins. They enjoy the results as divine nectar, and enter the eternal spiritual nature.

31

Arjuna, without sacrifice you cannot live happily in this world or the next.

32

These ways of sacrifice are laid out by the Vedas. They all arise from action: know this and you will be free.

33

Better than sacrifice of material possessions is sacrifice in knowledge, for work culminates in knowledge.

THE SYMBOLISM OF THE VEDIC FIRE CEREMONY, in which oblations such as ghee and grains are offered into the flames, is used in these verses. The fire represents the Supreme Being, and the oblations represent the fruits of work. This ritual is performed by Hindu priests, but Krishna extends its symbolism to all walks of life, saying that any work done in the spirit of sacrifice is as good as the sacred fire ceremony. Thus with mindful action the whole world and all work within it become sacred.

Krishna describes types of sacrifice: to the *Devas* who supply the necessities of life, such as water, heat and light; to the impersonal *Brahman*, sacrificing one's own identity; hearing and chanting sacred mantras; restraining sensual life; practicing the *astanga* yoga system (the eightfold path of mysticism taught by Patanjali, which includes meditation with focused vision and controlled breathing) to raise the consciousness; or *hatha* yoga to discipline the mind and body; fasting; pilgrimage; and studying scripture. Through such activities human life offers a route out of the material world for those who wish to take it. Though there are many kinds of happiness in this world, all of them bind the soul to the cycle of birth and death. Surpassing them is the happiness of the liberated spirit.

GIFT OF KNOWLEDGE

34

Learn from the wise with submission, inquiry and service. The self-realized souls who have seen the truth will give you knowledge.

35

Once you have received the truth you will never again fall into illusion, and you will see all living beings in me, the Self of all.

36

Even if you are the worst of all sinners, the boat of knowledge will carry you over the ocean of miseries.

37

As a blazing fire turns wood to ashes, so the fire of knowledge burns to ashes all karmic reactions.

38

In this world nothing is so pure as knowledge. In time the mature mystic discovers this knowledge from within.

39

A faithful person, dedicated, with senses subdued, soon achieves knowledge and attains transcendental peace.

40

An ignorant, faithless and doubting person is lost. The doubting soul cannot find happiness in this world or the next.

41

One who through yoga renounces action, whose doubts are
dispelled by knowledge, who lives in the self, is not bound
by work.

42

Therefore, Arjuna, with the weapon of knowledge remove
the doubts in your heart. Armed with yoga, stand and fight.

KNOWLEDGE IS THE KEY, AND THE WAY to acquire it is to listen with
humility to those who have seen the truth. This is Krishna's
advice. We cannot doubt everything and be happy. Faith in a
superior source of understanding is essential to find happiness.

If we put our trust in the scriptures and seek out those who
live their messages, personal association with such souls will
bring the scriptures to life. As Krishna says at the beginning of
this chapter, the knowledge of yoga was treasured and passed
from one king to another in exactly this way, and continues to
be passed on by the Lord's devotees living in this world.

If you cannot find the company of an enlightened soul, then
place your trust in Krishna. By reading his words in the *Bhagavad
Gita* you are hearing directly from your inner guide, who is with
you all the time. Krishna is the air we breathe, the space through
which we converse, the sense of touch by which we reach out
to one another. He is the Self within all, and by knowing him
we are in touch with all beings everywhere. To know Krishna
is the aim of life. Krishna is the boat to carry us over the ocean
of miseries.

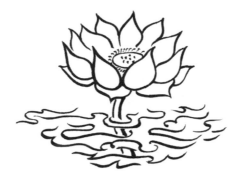

5

LIFE OF FREEDOM

As a lotus sits upon the water without becoming
wet, so the soul illuminated by wisdom lives in
this world in freedom and joy. The wise see all
beings as equal and the Lord as the friend of all.

FREEDOM THROUGH WORK

1

Arjuna said:

Krishna, first you recommend renouncing work, then work in yoga. Tell me clearly which is best.

2

The Blessed Lord said:

Renouncing work and work in yoga both lead to liberation. But of the two work in yoga is better.

3

The true renouncer feels neither hatred nor desire, and freed of these dualities easily escapes bondage.

4

The ignorant speak of yoga as different from the contemplative path. Yet a true follower of one of these paths achieves the results of both.

5

The position reached by the contemplative can also be reached by the one who works in yoga. One who sees contemplation and action as the same, truly sees.

6

Without the practice of yoga, renunciation is difficult. But a thoughtful person devoted to the practice of yoga soon achieves the Supreme.

7

A pure soul devoted to the practice of yoga, who controls the mind and senses, whose self is united with all selves in the Supreme Self, though always working, is not entangled.

KRISHNA HAS EXPLAINED THAT WORK in knowledge is called inaction, or *akarma*, because it is without karmic reaction. Now Arjuna asks for further clarification.

To practice yoga is to seek closer union with God. The essential point here is that the attempt to renounce the world will succeed only if we positively attach ourselves to God by acting in the awareness of God's presence. Yoga is more than theory. It is practical action.

Contemplation means to find Krishna as the root of the world. Having found the root, yoga waters the root. One who sees all beings as part of God loves all and is loved by all. By watering the root, the leaves and branches are nourished.

ENLIGHTENMENT

8

A person in divine consciousness sees, hears, touches, smells, eats, moves, sleeps and breathes, while all the time thinking, 'I do nothing.'

9

For speaking, evacuating, receiving, and opening or closing the eyes are only the interactions of the senses with their objects.

10

As the lotus leaf is untouched by water, so one who works without attachment, devoting all actions to the Lord, is untouched by sin.

11

Abandoning attachment, followers of yoga use their body, mind, intelligence and senses for self-purification.

12

One in divine consciousness lets go of the results of work and finds unbroken peace. The faithless one attached to the fruits of work is bound by desire.

13

The soul who mentally gives up all actions, doing or causing nothing, lives peacefully as ruler of the city of nine gates.

14

This ruler of the body does not create actions or cause their fruits, or induce others to act. All is done by nature.

15

The all-pervading Supreme Spirit is not responsible for the sinful or pious actions of the living beings. They are bewildered because their understanding is covered by ignorance.

16

As the sun lights up everything in the daytime, knowledge dispels ignorance and reveals everything.

17

When your intelligence, mind and faith take refuge in the Supreme, knowledge will cleanse away all your misgivings, and you will pass beyond the land of rebirth.

KNOWLEDGE REMOVES THE ILLUSION of material life to reveal the self as pure soul, different from the body and united with all life in the Supreme Lord. Such awareness illuminates everything and brings peace. Even though we may be active in so many ways, if our actions are dedicated to God they bring freedom.

The body is a gift of God. As long as we identify with this city of nine gates (eyes, nostrils, ears, mouth, anus and genitals) we are bound by it. But as soon as we identify with the Lord, who also dwells within the body, and use the body in his service, we are free.

The Lord is the constant companion in our heart. He perceives our desires without interfering with them, as a person smells the perfume of a flower without physical contact. He is impartial, and even though we are in illusion he does not deny us independence. Instead he helps us fulfil our desires in such a way as ultimately to bring us nearer to him.

SEEING WITH EQUAL VISION

18

The wise see with equal vision a learned and gentle priest, a cow, an elephant, a dog and an outcaste.

19

Those whose minds are balanced and even have already overcome rebirth. They are flawless like Brahman and therefore exist in Brahman.

20

A person who neither welcomes the pleasant nor rejects the unpleasant, who is self-intelligent, unbewildered, and knows the science of God, is situated in transcendence.

IF WE LEARN TO SEE ALL BEINGS AS DIVINE, as part of the Supreme, and therefore intimately connected with one another and with ourselves, we do not discriminate on the basis of species or form, or on the basis of caste, color or creed. The Lord himself is the friend of every creature, dwelling inside their hearts and treating them equally without discrimination. If we can understand this we also will feel friendship toward every being. Creatures who are less intelligent or weaker than us are even more deserving of our friendship. An enlightened person avoids giving pain to any animal, even to the smallest insect.

THE SOURCES OF MISERY

21

A person unattracted to external pleasures, who finds happiness within, is absorbed in the Supreme and enjoys unlimited bliss.

22

Pleasures arising from the senses are sources of misery. They have a beginning and an end, Arjuna, and the wise do not delight in them.

23

One who withstands the urges of desire and anger while living in this body is well situated and happy in this world.

SENSORY PLEASURES ARE DESCRIBED here as sources of misery. Sense enjoyment in a moderate way is a healthy part of life. But it is wise to control the body's sensory demands because sense pleasures are addictive and the cause of much misery.

The first step to spiritual consciousness is to know oneself as spirit, different from the body. As we overcome the illusion of being the physical body we can cultivate a steady mind unaffected by hatred and attraction. A steady mind does not rejoice at gain or lament at loss.

Of all pleasures in this world, sex is the most sought after. Sex is the motivation, conscious or otherwise, behind most of what goes on in human society, both the pleasure and the pain. If we can avoid being slaves to it we will avoid much suffering. We are set apart from animals by our ability to choose spiritual realisation, which is superior to material pleasure. The aim of human life is therefore to pursue self-knowledge and discover the bliss of the soul.

LIBERATION

24
One whose happiness and joy are within, who is illumined within, is liberated in the Supreme and attains Brahman.
25
Sages devoted to the welfare of all living beings, freed from sins, finished with doubts and with minds subdued, enter Brahman.
26
Ascetics freed from anger and desire, who are self-realized and self-disciplined, soon enter Brahman.
27–28
Excluding outward sensations, with gaze fixed between the eyebrows—with inward and outward breaths suspended within the nostrils, with senses, mind and intelligence under control—the contemplative, intent on liberation, is freed from desire, fear and anger and is forever liberated.
29
One who knows me as the enjoyer of all sacrifices and austerities, as Supreme Lord of all creation and as the friend of all beings, attains peace.

THE BLESSED STATE OF *BRAHMA-NIRVANA* is described here three times as the goal of sages and ascetics. It means to enter *Brahman*, to merge oneself into the Supreme Spirit. Some wish for their self, like a drop of water, to dissolve into the ocean of the Supreme and cease to exist as an individual. They are advised to practice *astanga* yoga, the eightfold path of mysticism taught by Patanjali, which includes meditation with focused vision and controlled breathing.

Devotees of Krishna do not aspire for this passive state of spiritual existence. They want to realize their eternal individuality as souls united with God through love, to realize their oneness with *Brahman* by entering an eternal spiritual relationship with the Lord. The first step toward this oneness is to practice Krishna consciousness—remembering the Lord. When this remembrance becomes constant all miseries fall away because the soul is immersed fully in the Supreme.

The real cause of suffering in this world is forgetfulness of the Supreme Friend. Those who are devoted to the welfare of all living beings try to revive Krishna consciousness in human society.

In concluding this chapter, Krishna summarizes knowledge: to recognize his presence throughout creation as the enjoyer, the friend and the goal of all our sacrifices in karma yoga. Since we all exist within the Supreme Lord we cannot enjoy this world without him. All peace will be ours when we know the One who is our supreme and innermost friend.

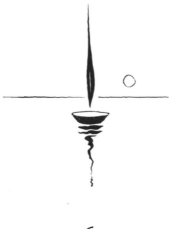

6

MYSTIC YOGA

Yoga leads to a still mind, steady like a lamp
in a windless place. The mystic who sees God
in all things is never separated from him and
is the perfect yogi.

GIVING UP SELFISH MOTIVATION

1

The Blessed Lord said:
One who works as required, without attachment to results,
is truly renounced and is a yogi—not one who gives up work
and worship.

2

Renunciation is the same as yoga, for yoga requires one to
give up selfish motivation.

3

For a beginner in yoga, the path is work; for one advanced in
yoga, the path is stillness.

4

One who abandons selfish motivation in sense enjoyment
and action is elevated in yoga.

KRISHNA ENCOURAGES THOSE WHO CARRY on with their lives,
doing as they are called to do, not drawing attention to themselves for the sake of recognition or profit, but working without attachment for the sake of goodness alone. These are the
silent yogis who live in the midst of every community, whose
relationship with God is more intimate than those who make a
show of prayer or meditation, or of abandoning the world.

Success in yoga depends on inner motivation and state
of mind. While being outwardly busy and active one may be
inwardly still. The popular practice of yoga starts with physical exercises, meant to lead to inner stillness. In the beginning
work alone is the means. Then gradually, through work, inner
stillness establishes itself within the mind. There Krishna is to
be found.

This state of inner stillness, or desirelessness, can be achieved by understanding ourselves as part of the complete whole of all existence. No one is independent from the web of life, materially or spiritually. Our interests are best served by working for the sake of the whole. One who sees the presence of Krishna in all of life sees all activities connected to the Supreme. The interest of the whole is served by working for the satisfaction of Krishna. This brings satisfaction to all the parts. When we experience fulfilment by this method, we no longer need to chase selfish desires or ambitions. We have achieved yoga: union with God.

MAKE THE MIND YOUR FRIEND

5

Let your mind elevate you, not degrade you. Your mind can be your friend as well as your enemy.

6

If you subdue your mind, it is your friend; but if you fail to do so, it behaves as your enemy.

7

One with subdued and tranquil mind lives in the company of the Supreme Self, whether in happiness or distress, heat or cold, honor or dishonor.

8

One who is satisfied through knowledge and realisation, whose senses are subdued, is established in yoga and sees earth, stone and gold as the same.

9

An elevated person looks on friends, enemies, relatives, colleagues, strangers, saints and sinners—all as equals.

THE FOUNDATION OF YOGA IS CONTROL of the mind. First we must learn to distinguish between ourselves and our mind. The mind is an instrument that can be used for both good or ill. A mind accustomed to obeying the demands of the senses leads to entanglement in material life. The normal function of the mind is to accept or reject, so it must be trained to accept beneficial things and reject harmful things. By training, the mind will gain a taste for pure foods, improving books, inspiring entertainment, enlightened company, and ultimately for service and devotion to God.

If the mind is clear of distractions it will naturally be governed by Krishna, and be the true friend and bringer of freedom. This is because it will not obscure the messages of the Supreme Self received within the heart. A clear mind, undistracted by the senses, is like a well-tuned radio receiver: it receives and communicates, free of background interference, the messages of God. One whose mind is tuned to this divine signal is always guided by the Lord.

When we recognize Krishna to be the essence of all we see the value in all, because all is part of Krishna. Consequently we lose the inclination to condemn others for their actions, for we know that Krishna permits all to act as they desire without condemnation.

HAPPINESS OF THE YOGI

10

The yogi, living alone in a secluded place with carefully controlled mind, free from desires and feelings of possessiveness, concentrates the whole self on the Supreme.

11–12

Practice yoga seated firmly on kusha grass covered by deer-skin and cloth, in a sanctified place not too high or too low. Control the senses and fix the mind on one point to purify the heart.

13–14

Hold the body, neck and head erect, gaze steadily at the tip of the nose, and with tranquil and subdued mind remain celibate and without fear. Thus meditate on me and sit absorbed in me as the highest goal of life.

15

Constantly absorbing the whole self in this way, the yogi of controlled mind reaches the supreme peace called *nirvana*, and lives with me.

16

Yoga is not for one who eats too much or too little, who sleeps too much or does not sleep enough.

17

One who is moderate in eating, sleeping, working and recreation banishes all sorrow through yoga.

18

One whose thoughts are restrained and rest in the self, free of all cravings, is established in yoga.

19

As a lamp in a windless place does not waver, so the yogi whose mind is controlled is steady in meditation on the self.

20

One whose mind is stilled by practice of yoga sees the self through the pure mind and rejoices in the self.

21

Reaching this state, one experiences boundless happiness through transcendental senses and never leaves the truth.

22

Having gained this place one imagines no greater gain, and is unmoved even by great misfortune.

23

This perfect state, untouched by suffering, is called yoga.

24

Practice this yoga with unwavering faith. Completely forsake all other aspirations and control the senses from all sides with the mind.

25

Step by step, using firm intelligence, withdraw into trance. Fix the mind on the self alone and think of nothing else.

26

Wherever the mind wanders because of its flickering and unsteady nature, bring it back under the control of the self.

27

Thus with mind at peace, with passions calmed, and freed from the burden of past deeds, the yogi gains supreme happiness and realizes Brahman.

28

Freed from all blemishes, the yogi who constantly practices yoga in this way easily achieves unlimited bliss in touch with the Supreme.

NOT EVERYONE CAN PRACTICE THIS SYSTEM of mystic yoga; but the basic principles set out here, such as fixing the mind on Krishna, controlling the senses, and following the path of moderation, are helpful to all kinds of yoga practice.

Nirvana means the end of illusion and the death of the illusory self. This is not the end of everything, for as the false self dies the eternal soul experiences the boundless joy of the soul's own spiritual nature. This joy culminates in the experience of union with God, in which the soul chooses to live eternally in love with Krishna. This is the eventual fruit of all yoga practice, whether it be the eightfold system of *astanga* yoga taught by Patanjali and described in this sixth chapter, or the devotional path of *bhakti* yoga taught by Krishna throughout the *Bhagavad Gita*.

For all who aspire to union with God there is an appropriate path that will suit. For example, one can follow the yoga diet of vegetables, fruits, grains and dairy products. These foods, combined in countless palatable recipes, simple or elaborate, when offered to Krishna with devotion, become sanctified. Their very essence is transformed by having been prepared in a spirit of devotion. As Krishna already taught in chapter 3, verse 13, these sanctified foods release their eater from all sins. Such food is itself enough to bring a person to the goal of yoga.

SEEING GOD IN ALL BEINGS

29

One absorbed in yoga, observing all beings equally, sees the Self in all beings and every being in the Self.

30

One who sees me everywhere and sees everything in me, never loses me and is never lost to me.

31

The mystic, who sees me as one in all beings, worships me with love and lives with me always.

32

One who sees oneself and all beings as equal, both in happiness and distress, is a perfect mystic.

GOD IS PRESENT EVERYWHERE THROUGHOUT the spiritual and material worlds. The difference between spirit and matter is a difference of vision only: one who can feel God's presence everywhere sees everything as spirit.

Every being is a particle of the Supreme Spirit, and the Supreme Spirit accompanies and guides every being. Because of forgetfulness we experience the illusion of separation from the Lord; but he is never separated from us, nor we from him. A mystic therefore offers love and respect to all beings, regardless of their outer appearance or status, knowing that the Lord lives in each of them as he does within one's own self, and that he favours them all equally, as a mother does her children. With this vision we understand that everyone, knowingly or unknowingly, serves God at all times.

THE RESTLESS MIND

33
Arjuna said:
This yoga of equanimity you have taught seems unendurable for the restless mind.
34
For the mind is turbulent, strong and obstinate, Krishna, and to subdue it is as difficult as controlling the wind.
35
The Blessed Lord said:
Truly the wayward mind is hard to subdue, but with practice and dispassion it can be trained.
36
For one with uncontrolled mind, yoga is hard to attain. Yet I say that with practice, one who strives with disciplined mind can succeed.

THE SOLITARY PRACTICE OF YOGA as Krishna has described above is, in this day and age, possible for only a few rare souls. There is no record even of Arjuna having attempted it. If it was difficult in his day, it is surely even more difficult today, when modern conditions create so many intrusions to distract the mind and senses, and when we lack spiritual training from an early age or widespread support in the community for this kind of spiritual quest.

Yet still Krishna recommends that with practice the mind can be controlled. The best way to begin controlling the mind is by hearing from a teacher who knows Krishna. By hearing about Krishna one will gain attraction for him and lose attachment to material things.

With the help of such a teacher one can bring the mind under the control of the intelligence. It is said in the *Upanishads* that the self is a passenger in the chariot of the body, which is pulled by five horses that are the five senses. Intelligence is the driver, and the mind is the reins controlling the horses. One whose intelligence keeps a firm hold over the mind, and so controls the senses, will be at peace and make progress in yoga.

The easiest way to control the mind in this age is to fix it on the sound of the Hare Krishna mantra, the great mantra for deliverance. This will place our minds with humility at the lotus feet of Krishna. If this is accompanied by eating food offered to Krishna, the mind will be pacified.

THERE IS NO SPIRITUAL FAILURE

37
Arjuna said:
What is the fate of a person who begins on the path of yoga with faith but who loses determination and falls away, failing to achieve success?

38
Is not such a person, bewildered on the path to transcendence, lost to either world like a fragment of cloud that evaporates in the vastness of the sky?

39
This is my doubt, Krishna, and you are the only one who can remove it. Please dispel this doubt completely.

40

The Blessed Lord said:

A person of faith is not lost in this world or the next. One who does good, my friend, is never overcome by evil.

41

One who falls from the path of yoga enjoys countless years in the heavens of the pious, and is then born on earth in a good and fortunate family.

42

Or one is born in a family of transcendentalists full of wisdom. Such a birth is hard to find in this world.

43

There one's former divine consciousness is reawakened and one strives further toward perfection.

44

This spiritual seeker, carried effortlessly onward by the influence of former practice, passes beyond the conventions of religion.

45

Thus with sincere effort the yogi is purified and perfected through many births, and at last achieves the supreme destination.

46

A yogi surpasses those who practice penance, or learning or ritual. Therefore, Arjuna, be a yogi.

47

Of all yogis, one whose innermost thoughts dwell in me, who faithfully serves me with devotion, I consider to be the greatest.

ONE MAY FORGO THE ILLUSION of material security in order to serve God, and then fall away from one's spiritual path, being apparently lost both to the spiritual and material worlds. Whereas material progress is lost with the end of this life, spiritual progress is never lost, even after many lifetimes. The path of spiritual growth continues from one lifetime to another. Therefore spiritual endeavors, no matter how incomplete, are never in vain. As soon as a soul expresses the desire to know Krishna, the universe responds to the soul's awakening search for the Supreme. From one lifetime to another the soul continues on the path back to Godhead, helped by the Lord and by the guides he sends.

Such souls, being already on the spiritual path, are naturally attracted to chanting the names of the Lord. They may appear uninterested in the outward formalities and rituals of religion, but once attracted to the lotus feet of the Lord, they do not forget his beauty and his mercy, and he does not forget them.

In the first six chapters of the *Bhagavad Gita* Krishna surveys the yoga path. This begins with karma yoga and progresses to include *jnana* yoga, the yoga of knowledge, and *dhyana* yoga, the yoga of meditation. Now, at the end of the opening section, Krishna concludes that *bhakti* yoga, devotional service to the Supreme Lord, is the culmination of all forms of yoga. In later chapters he will describe in detail the principles and practice of *bhakti* yoga.

PART TWO

THE MYSTERY
OF GOD

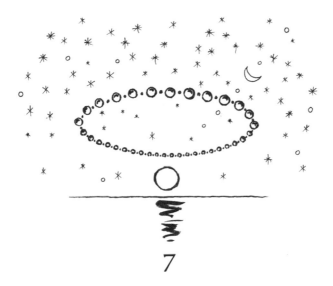

7

GOD AND HIS ENERGIES

Krishna teaches deeper knowledge. He is the
light of the sun and moon, the taste in water.
The worlds depend upon him as pearls strung
on a thread. A rare soul surrenders to him and is
released forever from birth and death.

RARE KNOWLEDGE

1

The Blessed Lord said:
Hear now, Arjuna, how by practicing yoga with your mind attached to me, making me your shelter, you can know me in full beyond all doubt.

2

I will teach you such knowledge and deep wisdom that there is nothing more for you to know.

3

Among thousands, one may strive for perfection, and of those who achieve perfection hardly one knows me in truth.

UNTIL NOW KRISHNA HAS TAUGHT about the self and the techniques to realize the self through different forms of yoga. He ends the sixth chapter by saying that the one who meditates upon him and serves him with devotion is the best of all followers of yoga.

Spiritual seekers who are not ready to take this leap of faith can follow the various paths of yoga outlined so far. For those who are prepared to place their full trust in Krishna he will now speak about himself and his energies.

The information given from here on is not available elsewhere. We may speculate about the nature and existence of God; but until we hear in faith directly from God himself we will remain in doubt. Most people are absorbed in experiencing material life and do not find time for understanding God. Even among those who seek to know him, God is hard to know unless we have faith to hear his words.

GOD'S ENERGIES

4

My material energies are divided into eight: earth, water,
fire, air, ether, mind, intelligence and ego.

5

Besides this external nature is my internal nature, made of
the living beings who sustain this world.

6

All are born from these two natures. I am the origin of the
entire universe and its dissolution too.

7

There is no truth superior to me. All rests on me as pearls
strung on a thread.

REALITY IS MADE OF GOD'S ENERGIES. The material world is formed
of his external energy, which is temporary, illusory, and sorrowful by nature. We conscious beings share the same nature as
God and belong to his internal energy, whose natural qualities
are *sat-chit-ananda*—eternity, knowledge, and bliss. The difference between ourselves and Krishna is that he is unlimited and
independent, whereas we are small and depend on him for our
existence, as sparks depend on a fire. God and the living entity
are one yet different.

GOD IS EVERYWHERE

8

I am the taste of water, the light of the sun and moon. I am
the syllable Om in the Vedas, the sound in ether, and ability
in human beings.

9

I am the original fragrance of the earth, the radiance in fire. I am the life of all that lives, the penance of all ascetics.

10

I am the seed of all beings, the intelligence of the intelligent, and the power of the powerful.

11

I am the strength of the strong, free of passion and desire, and I am desire that accords with the spirit.

12

The states of goodness, passion and darkness come from me and are within me, though I am not in them.

IF WE WISH TO SEE EVIDENCE OF GOD we have only to look around us and appreciate the wonders of this world. It is easy to take these wonders for granted: we can overlook the taste of water, for its taste is present in everything, as the sweet smell of earth is the basis of all perfumed flowers and aromatic forests. So it is with the presence of God. He permeates everything and so becomes invisible. All life is in him, yet it cannot contain him, for he is independent of all.

SEEKERS OF TRUTH

13

Deluded by these three modes of being, the world does not know me. I exist forever above them without change.

14

This divine illusion, created by me of the three modes, is hard to overcome. Yet those who seek my shelter pass beyond it.

15

Those who do harm do not seek my shelter: they are the foolish, the degraded, the bewildered, and the ones who have chosen the demoniac nature.

16

Among those who do good, four kinds serve me with devotion: they are the distressed, the seekers of wealth, the seekers of knowledge, and the wise.

17

Of these the wise, ever united with me in pure devotional service, are the best. I love them dearly, as they love me.

18

All these are noble souls, but the wise I consider as my own self, for they are absorbed in service to me, the ultimate goal.

THE MATERIAL WORLD EXISTS under the spell of Krishna's illusory energy called *maya*. Souls who choose to experience life without God enter the illusion of forgetfulness, and so God becomes hidden from them. Bound by the threefold ropes of illusion in the shape of goodness, passion and darkness, they enter various forms of life, pursuing their desires along never-ending paths.

MANY FAITHS

19

After many lifetimes, one in knowledge surrenders to me saying, 'Krishna is all.' Such a great soul is very rare.

20

Carried away by desires of all kinds, people give themselves to various gods and religious practices, according to their natures.

21

Whoever or whatever they choose for their faith and devotion, I encourage that chosen faith and make it firm.

22

With this faith they worship and obtain their desires, which in truth are granted by me.

23

Such rewards are temporary for those of small understanding. The worshipers of the gods go to the gods; my devotees come to me.

AFTER A LONG, LONG TIME spent searching for happiness in this way, a soul comes to understand that Krishna is all, and that there can never be any separation from him. Such a wise person at last surrenders to Krishna.

For those who choose to forget him, Krishna is never far away. He lives in the heart of every being in this world, giving us freedom to desire as we please, and helping us fulfil our desires. We are responsible for our choices, and for their consequences in the form of karma. Whatever it is we choose, Krishna encourages us on our path, ensuring we receive whatever we truly seek. He knows our desires better than we do, and responds to the deepest wishes of our souls. All paths lead eventually to him.

The gods referred to here are the *Devas*, or heavenly beings who govern the forces of nature, such as the planets and natural elements. Many powerful entities exist within the universe, far

God and His Energies

beyond the limits of our understanding. If we devote ourselves to the service of such beings we may be rewarded by them; even drawn in future lifetimes to live in the realms they occupy in the higher material spheres. Besides these are whatever gods we imagine for ourselves, based on our aspirations for security and happiness. All of these, real or imaginary, are extensions of Krishna. It is he who gives them the power to fulfil our dreams.

GOD IS HIDDEN

24

Those who do not know me think I am formless, though now dressed in form. They are unaware of my supreme nature, which is changeless and supreme.

25

I am not revealed to all, being hidden by my spiritual potency. This bewildered world does not know me, the unborn and imperishable.

26

I know the past, present and future of all beings, but no one knows me.

27

All beings who enter this world are born into delusion, bewildered by the dualities of desire and hatred.

28

Those who have acted well and put an end to harmful deeds are freed from these twin illusions and serve me with determination.

29

Those who take shelter in me, striving for release from old age and death, understand all about Brahman, the self and action.

30

Those who absorb their minds in me as the Supreme Lord, supporter of this world and its gods, and rewarder of all sacrifices, can know me even at the hour of death.

THE SOULS IN THIS WORLD are said here to be deluded by desire and hatred. These opposite emotions are akin to love and fear. Driven by these we inhabit an imagined world of opposites, desiring success and fearing failure, craving love and fearing rejection.

So long as we are caught in this web God's existence remains to us a mystery. Though he knows us intimately within our hearts—better than we know ourselves—still we cannot see him because we have chosen not to. As we become aware of our emptiness without him, and learn to pray and offer service to him, fear falls away. We can come to understand that in success or failure, in love or rejection, God is always with us.

Death is the moment of greatest fear. At that time when all that we know will be taken from us, our supreme good fortune will be to remember Krishna and accept his shelter.

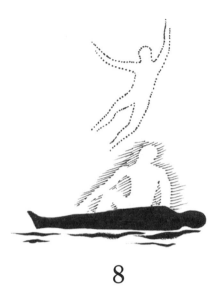

8

ATTAINING THE SUPREME

The onward journey of the soul depends upon
the state of mind at death. What we contemplate
becomes our future. One who leaves this world
remembering Krishna enters the eternal realm.

INGREDIENTS OF LIFE

1

Arjuna asked:

O Supreme Person, what is Brahman? What is the self and what is action? What is this material world and who are its gods?

2

How does the rewarder of sacrifices live in the body? And how can the self-controlled know you at the time of death?

3

The Blessed Lord said:

The imperishable soul, called Brahman, is the self. The evolution of living bodies is called action.

4

The ever-changing physical nature is called the material world. The gods and planets that make up this world are the visible form of the Cosmic Person, and I, the rewarder of sacrifices, live in the heart of all beings.

KRISHNA SPOKE OF HIMSELF at the end of the previous chapter as the supporter of the material world and its gods, and as the rewarder of sacrifices. He has also said that those who take shelter in him understand all about *Brahman*, the self and action, and that they can know him at the hour of death. Arjuna asks for more detailed knowledge about all this.

Krishna will speak more about these things and teach about what happens at the time of death and about the art of dying.

He will explain how he, as rewarder of sacrifices, lives in everyone's heart and fulfils all desires.

The Cosmic Person is conceived in the Vedic hymns in the form of the planets of the upper, middle and lower material realms and their controlling deities. This universal form of the Supreme Lord is contemplated by those who experience God in the sun and moon, in the oceans, and in the elements of nature.

HOW TO DIE

5

At the end of life, whoever departs the body remembering me attains my nature without fail.

6

Whatever nature you remember while leaving your body, that nature you will attain.

7

Therefore remember me always and fight on. With your mind and intelligence fixed on me, surely you will come to me.

8

One who meditates with constant practice and unwavering mind on me as the supreme divine person, is sure to reach me.

9

Think of me as knower of all, ancient, the ruler, smaller than the smallest, support of everything, of inconceivable form, beyond darkness, and radiant like the sun.

10

When death comes, with unwavering mind absorbed in devotion and strengthened by practice of yoga, those who fix the vital force firmly between their eyebrows reach the supreme divine person.

11

Ascetics who are free of passion practice celibacy so as to enter what the knowers of the Vedas call the Imperishable. I shall now briefly explain this path.

12

Closing the doors of the senses, focusing the mind on the heart and moving the vital force to the top of the head, you are established in yoga.

13

Vibrating the sacred syllable Om, which is Brahman, and remembering me as you depart this body, you will reach the supreme destination.

14

For those who remember me without deviation, Arjuna, constantly serving me with devotion, I am easy to obtain.

DEATH IS THE FINAL EXAMINATION which requires a lifetime of preparation. Whatever the mind remembers at death will create the pattern of our next life. We cannot all at once remember God if we have spent a lifetime forgetting him. The way our lifetime has been spent and the attachments we have formed in life will naturally occupy our mind at the approach of death. If we practice remembering God in the course of our lives, our minds will turn to him when death approaches.

Attaining the Supreme

This does not mean that we should give up ordinary occupations. Krishna does not advise Arjuna to stop fighting, rather to think of him while fighting. This is the basic principle of devotional service: to perform our duties in life while thinking of Krishna.

Death is a continuous process; at every moment the mind is called upon to die a little as the body nears its demise. It is best to be prepared at any time to leave this world. Saints advise that we live each day as if it were our last, keeping in mind the important things. It is easy to be complacent and forget the precariousness of life, as we are reminded when a friend or loved one is taken away without warning. Awareness of the mortality of the physical self does not mean to be morbid, but to remember and honor the immortal self as the intimate companion of God.

Constant remembrance of Krishna is called Krishna consciousness, and has the power to sanctify any place. We do not have to stay in a special sacred place, because service to Krishna can make anywhere sacred.

THE WORLD OF SAMSARA

15

Those elevated souls who come to me find the ultimate perfection. They never return to this fleeting place of sorrows.

16

The material worlds, even Brahma's heaven, are places of endless rebirth. One who reaches me is never reborn.

17

Brahma's day lasts a thousand ages and his night is of the same duration. Know this and you know the meaning of day and night.

18

In Brahma's dawn all creatures awaken; when night falls they once more merge into sleep.

19

Again and again the day comes and this host of beings is active; again the night falls and they are helplessly dissolved.

DAY AND NIGHT, LIKE BIRTH AND DEATH or youth and old age, are dualities of this world that remind us we do not permanently belong here. No one wants to die because the soul's nature is to live forever. Nor do we like change. We are creatures of security and familiarity. Yet this world forces change on us, and takes from us its comforts and assurances, driving us in our search for lasting peace. It is not a sign of weakness or inadequacy to want faith in something lasting. It is a recognition of the truth, that the ephemeral cannot satisfy the eternal soul. The best course is to live for God, and to love him in all we do and all we know. For he will never leave our side, and we will never lose his love—even when we lose this body.

Those who live good lives are rewarded in their next life. They may be reborn on earth in a pious or fortunate family, or they may be elevated to higher material realms. The highest such realm is *Brahmaloka*, the home of Brahma, chief of the gods of this universe. Souls remain in the heavenly realms for a long time—as long as their merit lasts. But eventually they fall back

Attaining the Supreme

to earth and the cycle of *samsara*, in which repeated birth and death continues. The only way to end this cycle is to be liberated through the practice of yoga.

THE ETERNAL WORLD

20

Above this dormant matter, hidden from view, is another eternal nature. When all in this world is annihilated, that part remains as it is.

21

That hidden place is called the imperishable and the supreme destination. Those who go there never return. That is my supreme abode.

22

The Supreme Person, in whom all beings rest and who pervades the world, can be reached by unwavering devotion.

THE SCRIPTURES OF THE WORLD TELL US about the abode of God, a place without death or anxiety, where love reigns supreme. Unless such a reality existed, generations of humanity would have felt no need to imagine it. If our nature were merely to die and be extinguished forever, we would not long for eternal life. The cause for this longing is that life is real and death is but an illusion.

REACHING THE SUPREME

23

Arjuna, I will now teach you when, passing from this world, the mystic either gains rebirth or does not return.

24

Knowers of Brahman, who pass away during the influence of the fire god, in daylight, in the bright phase of the moon, or in the six months when the sun travels in the north, go to Brahman.

25

Mystics who depart during the influence of the smoke god, at night, in the dark phase of the moon or in the six months when the sun travels in the south, after reaching the moon planet are reborn on earth.

26

These paths of light and dark are taught in the Vedas. One is the path of rebirth; the other the path of no return.

27

Yogis know these two paths, Arjuna, and are never deluded. Therefore be always fixed in yoga.

28

One who understands all this surpasses the merits earned by study of the Vedas, or by sacrifice, penance and charity. This yogi reaches the supreme original abode.

THE *BHAGAVAD GITA* CONTAINS in synopsis all aspects of Vedic wisdom, including this passage about the bright and dark paths.

The technique of passing from this world described here is meant for those with the power to choose their moment of death.

However, for one devoted to Krishna, every moment—bright or dark—is auspicious, since all is placed in Krishna's hands. All we need to know on the subject of dying has already been spoken by Krishna in the words, 'Remember me and you will come to my abode.'

As an aid to remembering Krishna one can chant the great mantra: *Hare Krishna Hare Krishna Krishna Krishna Hare Hare/ Hare Rama Hare Rama Rama Rama Hare Hare*.

This prayer occupies the mind, the tongue and the sense of hearing. It is the ever-present, direct and simple means to connect with God. Its regular practice is pure yoga, taking the place of all other spiritual disciplines.

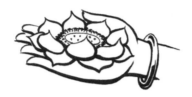

9

MOST CONFIDENTIAL KNOWLEDGE

Krishna is everywhere and all beings exist in him.
He calls for our love and offers us his support and
protection. If we give him a flower with love
he will accept it and release us from
the bonds of karma.

Most Confidental Knowledge

HEAR MY SECRET

1

The Blessed Lord said:
Arjuna, I will teach you the greatest secret because you are willing to hear me with trust. Once you grasp this knowledge and its application, you will be released from all miseries.

2

This secret is the summit of education, the innermost secret, the supreme purifier and the perfection of religion. It can be learned by direct experience, is easily and joyfully practiced and lasts forever.

3

Those with no faith on this path do not attain me. They return to the world of birth and death.

THE MORE WE ARE OPEN to hear from Krishna or from his devotee, the more he can teach us. What Krishna has to teach is the secret of life. If we know this secret, even the hardest experience can seem easy and joyful; without it the easiest thing becomes hard. Those who know the secret of Krishna consciousness appear to live, work and play like others. By living for Krishna they are gaining freedom; whereas those living only for themselves are prolonging their attachment to matter.

This secret is told to Arjuna because he is trusting and has opened his heart to Krishna. We must choose how we want to be. Life gives reasons not to trust others, and also reasons to show trust. Sometimes others fail us; at other times they give us hope. It is our choice whether to see our cup as half empty or half full.

The greatest question of trust is whether or not we are prepared to trust in a caring God. When things go wrong in life, I may be led to think there is no God, or God is unfair. But what appears to be misfortune may turn out to be good fortune in the long run. It can take a very long time to be in a position to know the full consequences of an act or an experience. One who trusts God even in difficult times, believing he is still there giving protection and love, has chosen trust and is a devotee of God. When we are baffled by life and unable to understand or control what is happening, we may be ready to let go and place ourselves with an open heart in God's hands. Then, as we open to God and to life, the secret of life opens to us.

Krishna calls the knowledge he now teaches *raja-vidya*, 'king of knowledge.' This is because this teaching summarizes all Vedic philosophies and is the essence of all wisdom. In particular, the king of knowledge deals with the inner nature of the soul and the soul's life beyond the confines of matter. Some believe that the soul, once liberated from the body, enters a passive state of oneness with God. Yet here Krishna describes this inner wisdom as eternally practiced. If the soul is eternal, then the soul is active eternally. The activities of spiritual reality are the subject of this most secret wisdom.

KRISHNA IS WITHIN AND BEYOND EVERYTHING

4

I pervade this universe with my hidden presence. All beings are in me, but I am not in them.

5

Yet all beings do not rest in me. Behold my mystic opulence: supporting all, yet beyond all, my Self is the source of everything.

6

See how the mighty wind, blowing everywhere, moves always within the vastness of space. So all beings move in me.

7

When one cycle ends, all beings enter my nature, and at the start of the next cycle I send them forth again.

8

Through my material energies I again and again send forth this host of beings. They are helpless in nature's embrace.

9

This work has no hold over me. I sit apart, detached from it all.

10

Under my direction nature produces all moving and nonmoving beings, and so the world revolves.

HERE BEGINS THE CONFIDENTIAL LESSON: Krishna is present everywhere, yet at the same time he is separate. This paradox is summarized by philosophers in the phrase 'inconceivable, simultaneous oneness and difference.'

Krishna is everywhere and we all live within him. Yet he is also beyond this world, untouched by the work of creation and maintenance. He is far away in the sense that he is detached and does not interfere.

Living beings have their desires, and at the beginning of each new cycle of creation he empowers them to go forth into the universal dawn to fulfil them. Krishna does not interfere in our freedom because he is generous and his nature is unlimited. He perfectly maintains this world, and still enjoys his own separate existence.

Krishna pervades the world, as the sun spreads its rays of warmth and light. At the same time Krishna is far away, as the sun is far away in the heavens. We can know Krishna partially by observing his material energies, but by thinking of him and becoming Krishna conscious we come to know him more. He has his personal existence and personal abode, and being the most loving person he reveals his personal existence to those who love him.

GREAT SOULS WORSHIP KRISHNA

11

The bewildered do not recognize me when I descend in human form. They do not know my transcendental nature as the Lord of all beings.

12

The hopes, work and knowledge of such misguided souls are all in vain, for their deluded nature attracts them to selfish and destructive ways.

13

Great souls seek the shelter of my divine nature. They know me as the inexhaustible origin of all beings, and serve me with single-minded devotion.

14

Always chanting my glories, endeavoring with great
determination, bowing down before me, these great souls
perpetually worship me with devotion.

WHEN KRISHNA DESCENDS TO EARTH HE reveals his personal
form and existence. Not everyone understands or believes that
Krishna has an eternal personal form. Some dismiss his form as
imaginary. Yet without God's personal existence and form we
see only half of reality. For the forms and personalities of this
world have their origins in the Supreme Godhead, whose form
and personality surpass all beauty.

A God who creates and maintains the material world and
rewards or punishes its inhabitants gives us every reason to obey
him, but little reason to love him. Krishna however does not
want our forced obedience. He wants us to choose freely to
love him. The great souls, mentioned here as always devoted
to Krishna, have understood that he is a loving person who
wants our love. Krishna eternally enjoys loving relationships
with his spiritual companions in a place beyond birth and death.
The most confidential knowledge of the *Bhagavad Gita* is that
Krishna invites us to join him there.

We are urged therefore to glorify Krishna continuously.
The essence of all religious practice is the constant glorification
of God. This is not just a formula for liturgical worship. It is a
continuous awareness of the unlimited grace of God working
in our lives to bring us to him. This requires us to cultivate that
mood of trust and open-heartedness already spoken of, looking
for the loving hand of God in everything, even in life's diffi-

culties. Inspired by this trusting mood, naturally we will praise him, thank him and love him for being there. This attitude turns every deed into an act of service to God. This is the meaning of the Sanskrit word *bhakti*, devotion; or as my teacher called it, 'devotional service.'

KRISHNA IS ALL

15

Others, who pursue knowledge, worship me as the One, as the many, or as the Cosmic Person.

16

I am the ritual. I am the sacrifice and the sacred gift. I am the healing herb and the holy chant. I am the butter, the fire and the offering into the fire.

17

I am father of the universe, mother, support and grandfather. I am what is to be known, the purifier and the syllable Om. I am the Vedic hymns: Rig, Sama and Yajur.

18

I am the goal, sustainer, master, witness, abode, refuge and most dear friend. I am origin, dissolution and foundation, the resting place and the eternal seed.

19

O Arjuna, I give heat and rain, and I withhold rain. I am immortality and I am death. Being and nonbeing are in me.

THESE ARE SOME OF THE WAYS KRISHNA can be worshiped indirectly. The worshipers of God as the One are monists who worship the self in all as one with God; the worshipers of God in the many worship the gods of the universe, such as the sun, moon and fire, as forms of the one God; and the worshipers of God in the Cosmic Form worship the entire universe as a form of God. For these last devotees, Krishna describes some of the ways that he can be experienced in the world.

These ways of experiencing God in the world allow us to remember him always. For example, we can experience the care and love of every mother for her child as a manifestation of Krishna. We usually call Krishna 'he,' but we may also call him 'she,' the mother. His female counterpart, Radha, personifies his mercy and love. Wherever he is, she is also. Without her Krishna does nothing. He is controlled by her love.

Rain is given by Krishna, yet he also withholds it. In the present day, with the growing threat of climate change, people might ask, why God should withhold rain, the most basic necessity of life. The answer has already been given in chapter three: rain depends upon the wheel of sacrifice, that is upon the cycle of giving and receiving. If humanity lives in harmony with nature's laws we will have abundance. The law of nature begins with the recognition that this world does not belong to us. It is lent into our care. Each of us may take our fair share, provided we give back in return. If, however, we take without giving, individually or collectively, we will have to accept nature's consequences.

FRUIT OF DEVOTION

20

Those who study the Vedas and drink soma juice worship me indirectly, seeking heavenly realms. Released from past sinful actions they earn merit and reach Indra's heaven where they enjoy godly delights.

21

After abundant heavenly pleasures their merits are exhausted and they return to this mortal world. They follow the Vedas to seek pleasure, so they remain in the world of birth and death.

22

For those who worship me with devotion, meditating on me alone, I bring what they need and preserve what they have.

23

Those devoted to other gods, who worship them with faith, worship me without full understanding.

24

They are unaware that I am the Lord and enjoyer of all sacrifice; therefore they fall.

25

The worshipers of the gods are born among the gods; worshipers of ancestors go to their ancestors; spirit worshipers join the spirits; and those who worship me come to me.

NO RELIGIOUS PATH IF FAITHFULLY PRACTICED is condemned in the *Bhagavad Gita*, which is broad in its acceptance of all paths of faith. Krishna receives all worship offered in good faith as indirect worship of himself.

Those who worship the powers of this world, in whatever form, can expect benefits; but these rewards do not last forever. The worshiper eventually falls and is reborn on earth in the cycle of birth and death.

Krishna promises to look after his devotees' welfare, materially and spiritually. No one need fear that by giving up material security to worship Krishna they will lack anything. Krishna will protect and maintain his devotees in such a way as to increase their faith in him.

GIVE EVERYTHING TO KRISHNA

26

If you offer me with love and devotion a leaf, a flower, fruit or water, I will accept it.

27

Whatever you do, eat, offer or give away, and whatever hardship you suffer—offer it to me.

28

Absorbed in this yoga of renunciation, you will be released from the bondage of actions and their results, pleasant or painful. Liberated, you will come to me.

TO PLEASE KRISHNA IS SIMPLE, because he will accept any offering when it is made with devotion, even a little water. On the basis of this revelation, devotees offer to Krishna whatever they eat. Vegetarian food prepared from vegetables, grains, fruits and dairy products can be offered to Krishna with prayers for him to accept such a humble offering. The food is thus spiritualized as *prasadam*, 'the mercy of God.'

Krishna encourages us to make all our eating an expression of love for God—to make any act, even our struggles, an act of devotion. Life's hardships are also opportunities to remember

God. It is easy to thank him for the good times; but the thanks we give him in the hard times, the struggles we offer him, show our faith and trust.

Life lived in this way frees us from karma. The cycle of karma is like a fruit-bearing tree representing actions which bear bitter or sweet fruits, experienced by us as reactions. These fruits in turn bear seeds, which lie dormant in our hearts as desires, waiting to grow into new trees of action. This unending cycle of karmic reaction is dissolved by daily devotion to the Lord. This means to work for Krishna, to think and plan how to serve the Lord, and to chant his name. This devotional service is so powerful that a single act of service can purify the heart, and so the truth is revealed.

A Devotee Never Perishes

29

I am equal to all: I reject none and I favour none. But those who serve me with devotion live in me, and I live in them.

30

Even one whose behavior is deeply harmful, but who serves me with faithful devotion, should be accepted as a worthy person of right intention.

31

This soul soon becomes righteous and attains lasting peace. Arjuna, boldly declare, 'My devotee never perishes.'

32

All those who seek my shelter, whatever their birth, gender, caste or status, attain the supreme destination.

33

How much more so those upright priests and saintly rulers who are devoted to me. Therefore, having come to this temporary world of suffering, be devoted to me.

34

Think of me always, become my devotee, worship me and bow down to me. Absorbed in me as your supreme goal, surely you will come to me.

KRISHNA LOVES US ALL UNCONDITIONALLY. He has no favourites. Yet his presence is more keenly felt by those who love him. So a personal exchange develops in which the Lord and the ones who love him respond to each other in a loving relationship.

God does not need to forgive anyone, because he does not take offense in the first place. No matter how a soul behaves, God loves each one, as a parent loves a child no matter what the child may do. His acceptance is so complete that he helps us even when our acts are selfish.

As the witness in each person's heart he has promised to fulfil our desires, and does so without prejudice. God's love is reason enough for us to accept not just those who serve him with devotion, but any child of his, without condemnation.

No one is barred from devotion to Krishna. The yoga principles set out a clear path of behavior; yet still a devotee may accidentally stray or be compromised by the demands of material existence. Anyone who chants Krishna's names or meditates on his form, regardless of that person's imperfections, is on the right path and worthy of love and respect. As such they will soon be freed from unwanted things and attain Krishna.

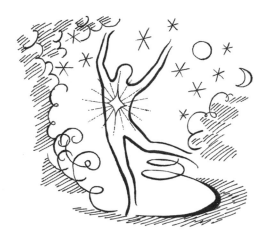

10

GOD'S INFINITY

Krishna is the origin of all and lives as the light
of wisdom in everyone's heart. Arjuna wishes to
know how the Blessed One can be perceived in
this world. In reply Krishna sings the poem of his
infinite forms.

KRISHNA'S SUPREME NATURE

1

The Blessed Lord said:

Listen further, my beloved, as I speak still higher knowledge for your benefit.

2

The gods and great sages do not know my origin, for I am the source of them all.

3

Whoever knows me as the unborn and beginningless Lord of all the worlds is undeluded among mortals and released from all sins.

4–5

Intelligence, knowledge, freedom from delusion, forgiveness, truthfulness, self-control, calmness, happiness, sorrow, birth, death, fear, fearlessness, nonviolence, equanimity, satisfaction, austerity, generosity, reputation and shame— these ways of being come from me alone.

6

The seven great enlightened ones and the four, along with the Manus, are born from my mind and share my nature. All creatures descend from them.

7

One who truly knows this opulence and power of mine is certain to find full absorption in yoga.

KRISHNA REVEALS SECRETS HIDDEN even from the gods To those who, like Arjuna, accept and return his love. These secrets can release us from our sins, which are like a chain of action and reaction unfolding from our past and imprisoning us. This release is possible because the force that binds us to our sins is not the condemnation of God, but our own attachment. We consider ourselves the independent cause of our actions, and so our attachments bind us and blind us to the possibility of freedom. If we learn to see our experiences not as our own, but as gifts of the Creator, we are free.

Krishna claims the good and the bad that we see in ourselves—our happiness and generosity as well as our fear and shame—as states of being manifested by him in response to our desires. When in our hearts we know the Lord of worlds as creator of our experiences and weaver of our dreams, we awaken from delusion and are relieved of the weight of karma.

The Vedic account of creation, referred to here in verse six, begins with the birth of Lord Brahma, the first created being. The beings listed are described in the Vedic literature as the primary beings in this universe, born directly from Brahma. They are the seven great sages who propounded the Vedic teachings; the four child sages known as the Kumara brothers, who do perpetual penance for the welfare of the universe; and the fourteen Manus who are the fathers of the human race and from whom descends the name 'man.'

HEART OF THE *BHAGAVAD GITA*

8

I am the source of all. Everything emanates from me. The wise who know this serve me with all their hearts.

9

With minds absorbed in me and lives surrendered to me, they enlighten one another and find deep satisfaction in speaking of me always, tasting transcendental bliss.

10

To those always absorbed in serving me with love, I give the understanding that leads to me.

11

Out of compassion for them, I dwell in their heart and destroy the darkness born of ignorance with the shining lamp of knowledge.

THESE FOUR VERSES ARE THE HEART of the *Bhagavad Gita*. Once the spiritual seeker has accepted Krishna as the source of all, faith and devotion naturally follow. Faith is nurtured in the company of Krishna's devotees, who find pleasure in discussing Krishna and his spiritual truths.

A devotee, with deepening faith, offers service to Krishna in body and mind. In response Krishna inwardly reveals that devotee's personal loving relationship with him. By the Lord's grace all obstacles are removed from the heart of the devotee who serves him.

The seed of devotional service to Krishna is sown in the heart by the mercy of Krishna's devotee. The seed is watered by regular hearing and chanting of Krishna's names. The plant of devotional service grows until it pierces the coverings of the material universe and enters the spiritual sky. There it penetrates the *brahmajyoti*, the dazzling spiritual effulgence, to find shelter in Goloka Vrindavan, the abode of Krishna, where it blossoms at Krishna's feet. In that stage a devotee is absorbed in hearing and chanting about Krishna at every moment.

ARJUNA'S PRAISE

12

Arjuna said:
You are the supreme spirit, the highest abode, the supreme purifier. You are the eternal, original divine person, unborn and all-pervading.

13

All sages say this of you, such as Narada, Asita, Devala, and Vyasa, and now you yourself are telling me.

14

I fully accept these truths you have given me, Krishna. Neither the gods nor demons understand your revelation.

15

You know yourself by your own power, O Supreme Person, Lord and Creator of all beings, God of gods, Lord of the universe.

IN THE PRECEDING VERSES KRISHNA delivers the essence of his message, offering himself in love to those who love him. Now Arjuna responds with his own affirmation, and he advances names of great Vedic teachers who have accepted Krishna's divinity.

The Vedic tradition carries spiritual authority in Asia, as have the wisdom traditions of the classical and biblical worlds in Europe. In the twenty-first century the teachings of East and West have become complementary parts of a common search for the divine shared by all peoples of the globe.

INFINITE FORMS OF GOD

16

Please tell me in detail of your divine powers by which you pervade all these worlds.

17

How shall I know you, Supreme Mystic, and always remember you? In what forms can you be contemplated, Blessed One?

18

Tell me again of your mystic opulences, for I never tire of hearing your sweet words.

19

The Blessed Lord said:

Yes, I will tell you my divine manifestations, the ones that are prominent—for my expansions are infinite.

20

I am the Self, seated in the hearts of all beings. I am the beginning, middle and end of all.

21

Of celestial deities I am Vishnu, among lights I am the radiant sun, of wind spirits I am Marichi and among stars I am the moon.

22

Of Vedas I am the Sama Veda, of gods I am Indra, of senses I am the mind and in living beings I am consciousness.

23

Of Rudras I am Shiva, of Yakshas and Rakshasas I am the lord of wealth, Kuvera, of Vasus I am the fire god, Agni, and of mountains I am Meru.

24

Of priests I am their chief, Brihaspati, of generals I am Skanda, god of war, and of bodies of water I am the ocean.

25

Of sages I am Bhrigu, of vibrations I am the syllable Om, of sacrifices I am japa, and of immovable things I am the Himalaya mountains, abodes of snow.

26

Of trees I am the peepal, of divine sages I am Narada, of the celestial singers I am Chitraratha, and among perfected beings I am the sage Kapila.

27

Of horses I am Uccaihshrava, born of nectar, of lordly elephants I am Airavata and among men I am the monarch.

28

Of weapons I am the thunderbolt, of cows I am the giver of abundant milk, of progenitors I am the god of love and among serpents I am Vasuki.

29

Of celestial snakes I am Ananta, of aquatics I am Varuna, of ancestors I am Aryama and among rulers I am Yama, lord of death.

30

Among demons I am the devoted Prahlada, of subduers I am time, of beasts I am the lion and among birds I am Garuda.

31

Of purifiers I am the wind, of wielders of weapons I am Rama, of fish I am the shark and among rivers I am the Ganges.

32

Of creations I am the beginning, middle and end, in education I am knowledge of the self and in argument I am the natural conclusion.

33

Of letters I am the vowel 'A' and among compound words I am the dual word. I am inexhaustible time and among creators I am Brahma, whose many faces turn everywhere.

34

I am all-devouring death and I am the source of all things yet to be. Among women I am fame, fortune, speech, memory, intelligence, constancy and patience.

35

Of hymns I am the Brihat-sama, of meters I am gayatri, of months I am Magasirsha, the month of harvest, and of seasons I am flower-bearing spring.

36

I am the gambling of cheats and the splendor of the splendid. I am victory, I am adventure and I am the strength of the strong.

37

Of descendants of Vrishni I am Vasudeva and of sons of Pandu I am Arjuna. Of the learned I am Vyasa and among great thinkers I am Ushana.

38

Among law enforcers I am the rod, among seekers of victory I am morality, of secret things I am silence and among the wise I am wisdom.

39

I am the generating seed of all beings. No being, moving or still, exists without me.

40

There is no end to my divine manifestations. These I have described give only an indication of my infinite opulences.

41

Know that all powerful, beautiful and glorious creations spring from but a spark of my splendor.

42

What need is there, Arjuna, for all these details? With a single fragment of myself I pervade and support this entire universe.

THE PEEPAL TREE, WHOSE SANSKRIT NAME is *asvattha*, is the most revered and long-lived of the fig family, which includes the banyan tree. Peepal and banyan trees are planted to give shelter to Hindu shrines. The peepal tree is also sacred to Buddhists because under it Gautama Buddha achieved enlightenment.

Japa is a simple method of prayer or meditation. A chosen mantra composed of names of God is repeated softly or silently while counting on a string of 108 beads called a *mala*.

This poem of the Universal Form gives us only an idea of Krishna's glories. If we examine any part of his creation we will find his wonders. As words carry the poet's thoughts, or music the mind of the composer, so the manifestations of nature in their endless variety, from smallest to greatest, display the infinite shades of colors, thoughts, energies, emotions and graces of Krishna, the supreme artist.

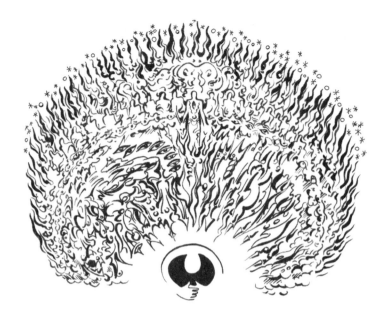

11

VISION OF THE UNIVERSAL FORM

Arjuna witnesses the awesome display of
Krishna's Universal Form, in which soldiers are
destroyed like moths in a flame. Filled with fear,
he prays to see Krishna's gentle form of love.

ARJUNA DESIRES DIVINE EYES

1

Arjuna said:

You have favoured me with this innermost spiritual secret, and your words have dispelled my illusion.

2

Lotus-eyed One, you have told me everything of the origin and destiny of living beings and your inexhaustible greatness.

3

As you have said, Lord, so you are. O Supreme Person, I wish to see your form of majesty.

4

If you think I have the eyes to see, Lord of Mystic Powers, show me your cosmic Self.

5

The Blessed Lord said:

Behold, Arjuna, my hundreds of thousands of divine forms, infinite in color and shape.

6

See here the Adityas, Vasus, Rudras, Ashvins, Maruts, and many wonders never before revealed.

7

See at once the entire universe, with all creatures moving and still, and whatever else you desire, here in my body.

8

But you cannot see me with your present eyes, so I give you divine eyes. Behold now my mystic opulence!

AFTER HEARING OF KRISHNA'S INFINITE energies Arjuna is convinced that Krishna is the source of everything. Now, for the sake of others, he wants Krishna to demonstrate his divinity. We naturally want to understand how God enters and supports the cosmos and we try through scientific research to penetrate the mysteries of reality. Such understanding, however, is limited to the human mind's capacity to receive it. Even if we could somehow see God's all-pervading presence we would be bewildered, as Arjuna is about to discover. The mind capable of holding such a universal vision is the mind of God.

KRISHNA REVEALS HIS UNIVERSAL FORM

9

Sanjaya said:

So saying, the Personality of Godhead, Supreme Lord of Mystic Power, revealed to Arjuna his Universal Form.

10–11

Arjuna saw numberless wonderful forms with countless mouths and eyes, clothed in celestial robes and garlands, adorned with divine ornaments and perfumes, and bearing many raised weapons. All were wondrous, effulgent, infinite and all-expanding.

12

If a thousand suns rose at once in the sky, their brilliance might equal the radiance of that Supreme Person.

13

In the body of the Lord of lords Arjuna saw the unlimited aspects of the universe united in one place.

14

Full of wonder, his hair raised on end, Arjuna bowed his
head before the Lord and prayed with folded hands.

ARJUNA'S VISION OF THE UNIVERSAL FORM is one of the great
mystical passages of world literature. It captures the majesty and
awesome power of the cosmic reality as well as can be commu-
nicated in words. There is more here than poetic fancy—these
words bear the authentic stamp of one who has witnessed at
least a fragment of what is described.

The spiritual seeker is sometimes blessed with a moment in
which the veil is lifted, allowing a glimpse of what lies beyond
the surface of normal life. These rare moments on the spiritual journey inspire faith and conviction. Yet they cannot be
sustained. Each of us must find in our everyday life the presence
of God. As Krishna has said in the sixth chapter, 'One who sees
me everywhere and sees everything in me, never loses me and
is never lost to me.'

AWESOME VISION

15

Arjuna said:

I see gathered in your body, Lord, gods and beings of all
kinds. I see Shiva, divine sages and serpents, and Brahma
seated on his lotus.

16

I see spread around me your limitless form with infinite arms, bellies, mouths and eyes. Lord of the universe, I see no beginning, middle or end to this cosmic vision.

17

Your dazzling form, adorned with crowns, clubs and discs, with fiery effulgence spread on every side, is hard to look upon like the sun.

18

You are the everlasting goal of knowledge, supreme shelter of the universe, enduring guardian of truth and the eternal Personality of Godhead. This is my conviction.

19

You have no beginning, middle or end. Your arms are numberless. The sun and moon are your eyes. Flames, blazing from your mouths, devour the universe.

20

The three worlds tremble, O Great One, to see your wonderful and terrible form consuming all space between heaven and earth.

21

Hosts of gods enter you, some in fear, offering prayers with folded hands. Saints and sages praise you. Crying, 'All peace!' they chant Vedic hymns.

22

The gods—Rudras, Adityas, Vasus, Sadhyas, Vishves, Ashvins and Maruts—along with forefathers, angels, spirits, demons and all perfected beings, behold you in wonder.

23

The worlds are terrified and so am I, by your vast form with infinite faces, eyes, arms, thighs, legs, bellies and fearsome teeth.

24

Seeing you spread across the sky, radiating infinite colors, with gaping mouths and great blazing eyes, my mind is lost. O Vishnu, I am afraid.

25

Lord of lords, refuge of the worlds, be merciful upon me. Seeing your blazing deathlike faces and mighty teeth I have lost all sense of direction and safety.

26

I see the sons of Dhritarashtra with Bhishma, Drona, Karna and their host of allies, and our heroes too, all entering your form.

27

They rush into your fearsome mouths, where some are caught with their heads crushed between your teeth.

28

As the waves of a river hasten to the ocean, so these great heroes enter your fiery throats.

29

As moths rush into the flames of a lamp, so all perish in your blazing mouths.

30

O Vishnu, your effulgence fills the universe and scorches all people. Thus your terrible radiance consumes all.

31

Lord of lords, so fierce of form, I bow before you. Please be merciful and tell me who you are. I wish to know you, Ancient One, and what your mission is.

THIS DISPLAY OF POWER fills Arjuna with fear. Fear of God is sometimes encouraged by religion because fear induces obedience. It is said that rulers of old used accounts of punishments in hell to frighten people into good behavior. Such forced obedience and fear may induce reverence and dependence on God, but it masks the true inclination of the soul. Fear must be replaced by love as the motivating factor in religion if the soul is to find happiness and if religion is to bring peace to the world.

THE VISION SPEAKS

32

The Blessed Lord said:

Time I am, destroyer of worlds, and I have come to destroy all beings. Except for you, all who enter this fight on both sides will be slain.

33

Rise, therefore, win glory, and after conquering your enemies enjoy the flourishing kingdom. They are already put to death by my arrangement, and you, Arjuna, can be but an instrument in the fight.

34

Drona, Bhishma, Jayadratha, Karna and the other great fighters are destroyed by me. Therefore, kill them without fear. Simply fight and you will vanquish your enemies.

EVENTS APPEAR ABHORRENT SOMETIMES, and God's will seems incomprehensible. At such times we can remember Krishna's words in the *Bhagavad Gita*. He urges us to have faith that the world moves to bring all souls to freedom and love when they are ready. God comes at last, even to the unfaithful, in the form of death, the ultimate fear in this world. One who seeks as Arjuna does to be God's instrument, living as Krishna has asked with detachment and compassion for others, has nothing to fear in life or in death.

ARJUNA'S PRAYERS

35

Sanjaya said:

Trembling with fear while hearing these words, with head bowed and folded hands, Arjuna praised Krishna in faltering voice.

36

Arjuna said:

The world becomes joyful hearing your name, Krishna, and all are attracted to you. Perfect ones revere you, but demons fly from you in fear.

37

And why should they not revere you, Great One? You are the infinite God of gods, original creator even of Brahma, and shelter of the universe. You are the imperishable cause of all, and yet you are beyond all.

38

You are the original Godhead, Oldest Person and highest abode of this universe. You are the one who knows and who is to be known, the supreme refuge. Your limitless form pervades the cosmos.

39

You are air, fire, water, moon and death, father and grand-father of all creatures. I offer my respects to you a thousand times, again and yet again!

40

I bow to you in front, behind and on all sides. Unbounded power, limitless might, you are everywhere and so you are everything.

41

Unaware of your greatness, I have in the past called you 'Krishna my friend,' in confusion and love.

42

I disrespected you, joking as we relaxed alone or with friends, lying on a bed, sitting or eating together. Infallible One, please forgive my offenses.

43

Father of all beings, worshiped by all as supreme teacher, no one in the three worlds can equal or surpass you, for your glory is beyond measure.

44

I fall to the ground imploring your mercy, worshipful Lord.
As a father with his son, as a friend with a friend, or a lover
with his beloved, be patient with me.

45

I see what has never been seen before, and I am grateful.
Yet my mind is full of fear. Please, therefore, show me your
own form and be kind to me, Lord of lords, refuge of the
universe.

46

O thousand-armed Cosmic Lord, I long to see your four-
handed form, with helmet on your head, and club and discus
in your hands.

KRISHNA HAS REVEALED TO ARJUNA that he will be successful in
the battle. Now, with nothing to fear, Arjuna is joyful. However,
those who act with hatred for others fear the power of God
because they fear the consequences of their actions. They do not
want to open their hearts to God or to anyone, for fear of expo-
sure and rejection. Thus they fear the very idea of God, from
whom there can be no secrets. This fear is groundless, because
God is the shelter of all and is merciful even to those who have
adopted the nature of demons.

Arjuna reminds Krishna of their personal friendship. This
means more to Arjuna than the display of Krishna's power as
Lord of the three worlds (the heavens, the earth and the lower
realms). Krishna's love for his devotees, as a father, as a friend,
or as a lover, is revealed in Krishna's play on earth. In such rela-

tionships Krishna's power and divinity is forgotten in the presence of love.

SEEING WITH THE EYES OF LOVE

47

The Blessed Lord said:

Dear Arjuna, I am glad to show you this supreme form through my mystic power. No one before you has seen this primal, infinite and dazzling vision.

48

This cannot be seen by study of the Vedas, sacrifice, charity, pious works or severe penances. You are the only one in this world to have seen this.

49

You have been troubled and bewildered by this frightening aspect of mine. Now let it be finished. With peaceful heart and without fear, see my own form.

50

Sanjaya said:

So saying, Krishna showed his four-armed form. Encouraging the fearful Arjuna, the Great One then resumed his gentle and most beautiful appearance.

51

Arjuna said:

Krishna, seeing your humanlike form, so gentle, my mind is pacified and I am restored to my original nature.

52

The Blessed Lord said:

This form of mine seen by you is very difficult to behold. The gods always long to see this form.

53

This form is not revealed through study of the Vedas, penance, charity or worship.

54

Dear Arjuna, you can know and see me as I am, here before you, only by undivided devotional service, and so enter the mysteries of my existence.

55

One who works for me in devotion, depending on me without worldly attachments, being friendly to all beings, comes to me.

KRISHNA'S MOST INTIMATE FORM is called here *saumyam*, meaning 'gentle and beautiful.' This form is unlike the majestic and frightening Universal Form, because it is intended for his loving relationships with his devotees. Krishna's four-handed form, requested by Arjuna, is his majestic form as Narayana, worshiped and served in reverence. After showing this Narayana form he returned to his intimate humanlike appearance as Govinda. This original form can be seen and understood by those who serve Krishna in devotion, giving up worldly association and showing love to others. Krishna with two hands playing the flute, dancing with his companions in the forest of Vrindavan, is the most personal vision of God. To see this form of Krishna is truly to enter the mysteries of his existence.

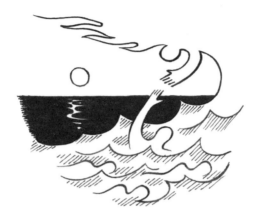

12

THE WAY OF DEVOTION

The path of personal devotion and the path of
impersonal meditation both lead to Krishna,
who rescues his devotees from the ocean of birth
and death. He recommends the path of personal
devotion and describes the qualities of those
who are dear to him.

SERVICE OR MEDITATION?

1

Arjuna said:

Some always serve you in devotion, and others contemplate the Imperishable and Imperceptible. Which are the most perfect in yoga?

2

The Blessed Lord said:

Those whose minds are focused on me, absorbed in my constant service with great faith, I consider the most perfect yogis.

3-4

Those who contemplate the imperceptible   the invisible, all-pervading, inconceivable, unchanging, fixed and immovable—who control the senses, are even-minded and live for the welfare of all, also attain me.

5

Yet their trouble is great, for the path to the imperceptible is difficult for mortals to follow.

6-7

Those who dedicate all their actions to me—who are attached to me and absorbed in yoga, who remember and worship me, whose minds are fixed on me—I soon deliver from the ocean of birth and death.

TWO SPIRITUAL PATHS ARE FOLLOWED by practitioners of yoga: the path of devotion and the path of impersonal contemplation. Ultimately both paths reach the same goal, but Krishna says at the end of the sixth chapter that one who faithfully serves him with devotion is the greatest yogi. Now Arjuna asks about those who are attracted to the all-pervading impersonal aspect of God.

Having witnessed the display of Krishna's inconceivable energies, Arjuna wants to be reassured that he really can enter a personal, devotional relationship with this Universal Lord. Is such a personal relationship real, or is it better to follow the other path, to contemplate the impersonal Oneness?

Krishna here distinguishes between the two paths. The path of personal devotion, *bhakti* yoga, is direct and most perfect; the path of abstract meditation, *jnana* yoga, also leads to perfection, but is difficult and troublesome. One path depends on the grace of the Lord and the other on the determination of the follower. Krishna's advice is clear: follow the path of devotion.

STAGES ON THE PATH

8

Fix your mind on me, absorb your intelligence in me. Thus you will live in me always, without a doubt.

9

If you cannot fix your mind upon me without deviation, then try to reach me by regular practice of yoga.

10

If you cannot do this regular practice, then devote yourself to working for me, for just by working for my sake you will achieve perfection.

11

If you are unable to work under my shelter, then control your mind and work without attachment to the fruits of your actions.

12

Knowledge is better than practice, meditation is better than knowledge, and giving up the fruits of action is better than meditation, for from detachment comes peace.

HERE ARE THE STAGES OF DEVOTIONAL practice in descending order. The highest stage is full absorption in spontaneous love for Krishna, through which every act merges into transcendence. The way to achieve this consciousness is to follow the principles of *bhakti* yoga under the guidance of a teacher. This will purify one's senses in the service of Krishna. This practice begins with hearing and chanting Krishna's names, associating with his devotees, and remembering him.

If this practice is not possible, you can serve Krishna by supporting his work and the work of his devotees, or by devoting yourself to Krishna in your occupation according your natural abilities.

At the same time you can chant *Hare Krishna Hare Krishna Krishna Krishna Hare Hare/ Hare Rama Hare Rama Rama Rama Hare Hare*.

If none of these methods is possible, you can practice karma yoga, giving up the results of your work for the welfare of others and ultimately for the Supreme.

For those not attracted to the path of devotional service, the Lord lastly summarizes the impersonal path that leads from action to knowledge, from knowledge to meditation, from meditation to detachment, and finally to peace and liberation from material life.

ONE WHO IS DEAR TO THE LORD

13

One who bears no hatred, who is a compassionate friend to all creatures, who is not possessive or selfish, equal in happiness and distress, and forgiving,

14

Who is dedicated to the spiritual path, always satisfied, self-controlled and determined, whose mind and intelligence are fixed on me—this devotee of mine is dear to me.

15

One who troubles no one and is troubled by no one, who is unmoved by happiness, anger, fear, or distress—is dear to me.

16

One who is detached, pure, skilful, without cares or troubles and selfless in all endeavours—this devotee of mine is dear to me.

17

One who does not grasp joy or hatred, grief or desire, good or bad—this devoted soul is dear to me.

18–19

One who looks equally on friends or enemies, honor or dishonor, heat or cold, happiness or distress, praise or blame, who craves nothing, is silent and satisfied in any situation, who has no home, who is even-minded and filled with devotion—such a person is dear to me.

20

Those who faithfully follow this eternal path of devotion, making me their Supreme Goal, are dearly beloved to me.

THE QUALITIES OF ONE DEVOTED TO THE LORD are the inner qualities of the soul, revealed as the spirit is progressively freed from the coverings of material ego. Such qualities are naturally attractive to the Lord. A devotee of Krishna accepts distress as a just consequence of distress given to others and as an opportunity to learn and purify the heart. By the Lord's mercy this distress is kept to a minimum and so the devotee is calm and quiet despite all difficulties. A devotee is kind to all creatures, even to those who consider themselves enemies, because the devotee identifies with the spirit, not the body. To be silent means to speak only the truth about Krishna and the spirit. To have no home means to feel equally at home under the sky or in a comfortable residence.

The theme underlying all these qualities is one of detachment and acceptance, and ultimately of surrender to the will of the Lord. It is said that there are six aspects of surrender to Krishna:

1. Accept all that is favourable to the Lord's service
2. Avoid all that is unfavourable to the Lord's service
3. Have full faith in the Lord as protector
4. Have confidence in the Lord as maintainer
5. Be dependent on the will of the Lord
6. Be always humble before the Lord

On the path of surrender to Krishna one feels increasing joy. Therefore the path is described by the Lord as *amrita*, 'full of nectar.' To have faith on the path of devotional service means to believe that simply by offering service to Krishna all other needs will be taken care of. The benefits that arise from all other paths—whether by penance, sacrifice, religious ritual, obedience, morality, duty or study—are all fulfilled by making Krishna the supreme goal of life.

The conclusion of the twelfth chapter is that the path of mystic meditation on the impersonal aspect of God is recommended so long as one's love for Krishna is dormant. By good fortune, when the soul hears about Krishna from a devotee, that dormant love of God is awoken. Then the path of devotional service opens and the devoted soul is soon rescued from the ocean of birth and death.

PART THREE

THE JOURNEY

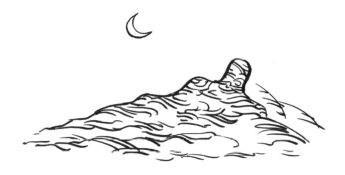

13

NATURE AND THE SOUL

The soul labors in the field of this body,
harvesting the fruits of happiness and distress.
Wisdom is to see the difference between the
field and the soul. Such wisdom is a gift of the
Supersoul who dwells within all beings.

THE FIELD OF ACTION

1

Arjuna said:

Krishna, I wish to know of nature and the soul, of the field of action and the knower of the field, and of knowledge and the end of knowledge.

2

The Blessed Lord said:

This body is the field, and the one conscious of it is the knower of the field. So it is said by the wise.

3

I am also the knower of the field in all bodies. To understand this field and its knower I regard as true wisdom.

4

Hear from me in brief about the nature of the field, its source and forms, and about the one who knows and influences it.

5

Sages have sung of this in various ways in the Vedic hymns, and analyzed its causes and effects in such writings as the Brahma Sutras.

6–7

These, in essence, make up the field and its forms: the five physical elements, ego, intellect, the total material substance, the eleven senses and organs with the mind, the five sensory objects, desire and hatred, pleasure and pain, the combination of all these, consciousness and conviction.

THIS WORLD IS A COMBINATION OF SPIRIT and matter. Spirit is eternal, active and joyful; whereas the forms of matter are

Nature and the Soul

temporary, passive and without feeling. When spirit and matter combine, the endless fluctuations and varieties of earthly life are produced.

The analogy of a field is given for the material body, because a field is where we labor to plant and nurture grains for the harvest, witnessed by the sun and rain. Similarly the soul, wishing to enjoy the fruits of work, labors in the field of the world amid the mind and senses, harvesting the fruits of happiness or sorrow, witnessed by the Supreme Lord. By realising ourselves as separate from the field we are freed.

The ancient philosophy called *Sankhya* analyzes the field into the twenty-four elements summarized here. The aim of *Sankhya* philosophy is to distinguish the soul from these twenty-four, which include the mind, intellect and ego. The soul is none of these, nor is it an illusion arising from interactions of molecules. It is eternal spirit distinct from matter. If we are truthfully to understand this world and the aim of life we must learn to distinguish between matter and spirit.

THE SUM OF ALL KNOWLEDGE

8–12

Humility, modesty, nonviolence, forgiveness, truthfulness, service to the teacher, cleanliness, steadiness, self-control, freedom from sensual desires, absence of false ego, awareness of the pain and sorrow of birth, death, old age and disease, detachment from the comforts of family and home, even-mindedness amid pleasant and unpleasant events, unwavering devotion to my service, attraction to secluded places, aversion to the crowd, dedication to self-realisation and pursuit of truth—these are said to make up knowledge. Whatever is contrary to these is ignorance.

THE FOUNDATION OF KNOWLEDGE is the realisation that the soul is different from the body. One who lives in the awareness of being a spirit in the material world will naturally incline toward humility, respect for all beings and detachment from material life. The more we understand, the less we find we know. Thus the sign of knowledge is humility. In time such understanding leads the wise to surrender themselves to the Supreme Lord, who is the end of knowledge described in the following verses.

THE END OF KNOWLEDGE

13
I will tell you the end of knowledge, by which you will taste eternity. This is called the beginningless Brahman, which emanates from me and lies beyond the cause and effect of this world.

14
Everywhere are his hands and legs, his eyes and faces, and he hears everything. In this way he covers the world.

15
He is the source of the senses, yet without senses. He is unattached and yet maintains all. He transcends the qualities of nature, and yet enjoys them.

16
He exists within and outside all beings, moving and still. He is far away, beyond the perception of the senses, yet very near.

17

He exists as one yet appears divided among all beings. He, the creator, maintainer and dissolver of all, is the end of knowledge.

18

He is the light of all that shines, beyond the darkness of matter. He is knowledge, the end of knowledge and the goal of knowledge. He dwells in everyone's heart.

19

This summarizes the field of activities, knowledge and the end of knowledge. My devotee who understands this attains my nature.

THE INDIVIDUAL SOUL AND THE SUPREME soul are both *Brahman*, or spirit, and they are described as the end of knowledge, the final truth. The individual soul in each body is called the *atma*, while the Supreme Soul, expanded as one soul inhabiting all bodies, is called in Sanskrit the *Paramatma* (Supersoul). The individual soul and the Supersoul are one in quality as pure spirit, but different in quantity. The soul is described in the *Upanishads* as infinitesimally small, one ten-thousandth the size of the tip of a hair. The Supersoul is infinitely large. The soul, being small, may forget the Supersoul, but the Supersoul never forgets the soul; they are never separated.

The Supreme is without material senses and qualities, but he possesses spiritual senses and qualities. He is the source of the senses and qualities of this world. Whatever exists in this world has its origin in him.

SOUL AND SUPERSOUL

20

Know nature and the soul to be beginningless, and nature as the source of the changing forms and qualities of matter.

21

Nature is the cause of activities and effects. The soul is the cause of feelings of suffering or enjoyment. So it is said.

22

Thus the soul, dwelling in nature, is attracted to nature's qualities and under their influence meets with good or bad fortune in different births.

23

The Supreme Soul is the Witness, living in all bodies as ordainer, enjoyer and sustainer. He is the Lord of all, called the Supersoul.

24

Those who understand this teaching of the soul, nature and the qualities of nature, regardless of their present state, will not be born again.

THE SOUL SEEKS ENJOYMENT because joy is the nature of spirit. This search leads the soul, through attraction to different qualities of nature, to be born in different wombs, fortunate or unfortunate, and to travel throughout the universe experiencing transient happiness and distress. This process of transmigration influenced by the qualities of nature will be described later.

The Supersoul, as ordainer and sustainer, supports the individual soul on this journey of experience and discovery, arranging for different bodies and senses to aid self-discovery and ultimately to bring the soul to true understanding. All the while the Lord as Witness speaks to us through our inner voice of conscience and wisdom. He speaks in dreams, through the mind or intelligence, through sacred books and teachers, and through the world around us. His guidance is always there if we are open to receiving it. The Supersoul is the enjoyer because he is the inspiration behind all enjoyment. Once we recognize him as our friend we will taste the joy of the spirit and no longer be attracted to rebirth in this world.

It is written in the *Mundaka Upanishad* (3.1.2) that God dwells beside the individual soul in the tree of the body:

'Two birds, inseparable friends, sit in the same tree. One eats the fruits while the other observes. The one who tastes the fruits, some bitter some sweet, is filled with anxiety and sorrow. If he turns to his friend, the Lord, and knows his glories, his grief comes to an end.'

Krishna is the Supersoul in person, who accompanies each one of us from one body to the next on our journey through the universe.

THE LIGHT OF WISDOM

25

Some see the Supersoul within through meditation, others through the path of knowledge, and others through the path of action.

26

Some, though they do not understand, hear with faith from those who do and so worship the Lord. They too pass beyond death.

27

Whatever exists in this world, moving or still, Arjuna, is a combination of the field and the knower of the field.

28

One who sees the Supersoul dwelling equally in all beings, everlasting amid the transient, truly sees.

29

One who sees the Lord equally present everywhere never harms the self, and so attains the supreme goal.

30

One who sees that all is done by nature, while the self does nothing, truly sees.

31

A person who sees the multitude of separate beings expanded everywhere, all existing in the One, attains Brahman.

32

The transcendent self, beginningless and imperishable, is beyond material qualities. Though dwelling in the body, the self does nothing and is unaffected by matter.

33

The sky, though everywhere, remains pure because it is subtle. Similarly the self, though inhabiting the body, is untouched.

34

As the sun illuminates the whole world, so the self, knower of the field, illuminates the field of the body.

35

Those who see by the light of wisdom this distinction between the field and its knower and see the path to freedom from matter, attain the Supreme.

THE LIGHT OF SPIRITUAL WISDOM reveals the Supersoul present in all beings, sustaining all and impartially witnessing our lives. With this understanding it is possible to accept all beings as they are—since the Lord himself does so—and do no harm to any creature, including ourselves. This way lies peace.

The soul illuminates the body with consciousness as the sun lights up the world. As the sun is untouched by the world, so the soul is untouched by the body and its actions. The soul does not control the body. It merely desires to act and the rest is done by nature. The body is controlled by nature under the direction of the Supersoul. We must therefore accept the limitations of the body we have been given and aim our desires toward the service of the Lord.

To those who cannot understand this thirteenth chapter of the *Bhagavad Gita*, Krishna gives encouragement in verse 26: if they hear these truths with faith from a spiritual teacher who understands them, they will still be freed from the cycle of birth and death.

The *Bhagavad Gita* is a scripture of grace inserted into the *Mahabharata*, the popular history of ancient India. It is intended to be heard and understood by ordinary folk who are not philosophers or renouncers of the world. Its message of grace is especially relevant in today's distracted world, where many have lost faith in religion. Krishna's path of grace grants spiritual knowledge not through learning or good behavior, but through devotion. If, by hearing with faith, we take to the worship of God—most easily by chanting his names—Krishna assures us of liberation from birth and death.

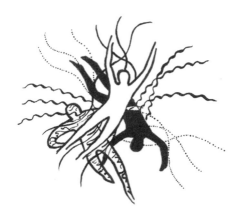

14

THE THREE QUALITIES OF NATURE

Nature is made of goodness, passion and darkness. These three qualities combine to produce all forms and actions. If you can be undisturbed by these qualities, and know that Krishna lies beyond them, you are free.

FATHER OF ALL

1

The Blessed Lord said:

I shall teach further supreme wisdom, the highest of all knowledge. The sages who understood this achieved supreme perfection.

2

By taking shelter of this knowledge one attains my own nature. Thus one is not born at the time of creation or disturbed at the time of dissolution.

3

Nature is the womb in whom I place my seed, causing the birth of all living beings, Arjuna.

4

All species born into this world come from the womb of nature, with me as their seed-giving father.

IT IS SAID THAT NATURE IS IMPREGNATED by the glance of the Lord, and from her womb are born all creatures, on the land, in the air, and in the waters, on this planet and on all other planets of the universe.

In this chapter Krishna, as father of us all, offers knowledge that goes beyond any he has taught so far. He reveals practical information about how material nature makes us behave the way we do. As children of nature and Krishna we are influenced by both mother and father. Mother nature's influence binds us to her and our divine father calls us to self-discovery. By understanding the three qualities of nature and how they act, we can become conscious of the way nature binds us. Then we can begin to change our behavior.

The same principle applies here as with the influences we receive in childhood from our parents. So long as we are unaware of our childhood conditioning we are bound by it; but by recognising it we have the option to change the way we act. Here, and in the following chapters, Krishna gives the tools for personal transformation, to enable us to change our habits from darkness and passion to goodness, and so discover our identity as pure soul.

Nature's Three Qualities

5

The primary qualities of goodness, passion and darkness, arising from nature, bind the eternal soul to the body.

6

The quality of goodness is purity, which brings illumination and well-being. Goodness binds the self with attachment to happiness and learning.

7

The quality of passion is desire, born of attraction and longing. Passion binds the self with attachment to work.

8

The quality of darkness is ignorance, which deludes all beings. Darkness binds the self with forgetfulness, laziness and sleep.

THE THREE PRIMARY QUALITIES OF NATURE are each called *guna*, which in Sanskrit means 'rope.' Goodness is *sattva guna*; passion is *raja guna*; darkness is *tama guna*. Woven together these three bind us to the world. As the three primary colors of yellow, red and blue mix to create all colors, the qualities of nature combine and interact in endless permutations. So long as we live in this world we cannot escape their influence. They affect all that we do.

HOW THE THREE INTERACT

9
Goodness gives rise to happiness; passion to work; darkness covers your knowledge and attracts you to forgetfulness.
10
Sometimes goodness prevails over passion and darkness, or passion dominates goodness and darkness, or darkness overwhelms goodness and passion.
11
When the light of understanding radiates through all the doors of the body, know that goodness prevails.
12
Greed, hard work, ambition, dissatisfaction and craving arise when passion dominates.
13
Depression, laziness, forgetfulness and delusion arise when darkness overwhelms.

14

A soul who passes from this world under the influence of
goodness attains the pure realms of the enlightened.

15

The soul who passes away in passion is reborn among those
attached to work. One who dies in darkness is born into the
animal kingdom.

16

The fruit of work in goodness is purity and more goodness.
The fruit of passion is unhappiness. The fruit of darkness is
ignorance.

THE EARTHLY REALM IS DOMINATED by passion, which urges
people to work and compete for success and power. Under the
influence of passion we seek a sexual partner with whom to set
up a home and gather possessions, so forming the foundation
for social and economic development. Passion carries a high
price: under its influence we are never satisfied and always want
more. This leads to struggles for supremacy between people,
communities and nations, both in business and in war. Nature
has provided enough for all her children, but human greed
creates constant competition for her precious resources. The
conflicts and human misery thus engendered are the product
of passion.

Goodness brings happiness and knowledge. A person
influenced by this quality is peaceful and self-sufficient, prefer-
ring not to compete with those in passion. But goodness binds
the soul to a false sense of satisfaction and security in an inse-
cure world.

Darkness brings forgetfulness and delusion. Where people have lost their sense of purpose, having no respect for themselves or others, taking shelter in intoxication to deaden their minds—there is darkness. In this condition the qualities of the soul seem to be negated, so that a person may behave in a way that is destructive or cruel. This effect of the quality of darkness will be examined in the sixteenth chapter of the *Bhagavad Gita*.

UNDERSTANDING THE THREE

17

From goodness is born knowledge; from passion comes greed; darkness brings forgetfulness, delusion and ignorance.

18

Those situated in goodness rise upward; those in passion stay in this middle realm; those ruled by darkness, lowest of all, sink downward.

19

One who sees no other performer at work than these primary qualities, and knows what lies beyond them, attains my nature.

20

The soul who rises above these three earthly qualities is freed from birth, death, old age and their distresses, and tastes the nectar of eternal life.

LIVING BEINGS MOVE CEASELESSLY UPWARD or downward through species and spheres of existence. The destination we reach in the next life is a consequence of our choices in this one. Human life on earth offers freedom to choose our future destination, either to return to this earthly realm of passion or to rise upward. Above the earth are heavenly planes where the enlightened proceed, or where souls are rewarded for their good deeds on earth. Beneath human life are the species of animal and plant life. If we live in darkness we deny our spiritual nature. In response to that choice the soul sinks into animal species where its spiritual nature is covered, or into the forms of plants or trees where the soul enters deep slumber.

In today's world the influence of passion and darkness are dominant. As a consequence we are laying down problems for the future in our lives and in the future life of the planet. The solution lies in cultivating the quality of goodness in all ways possible, as will be described in the remaining chapters.

TRANSCENDING THE THREE

21

Arjuna said:

What are the signs and behavior of one who has risen above the three qualities, Lord, and how does one transcend these three?

22

The Blessed Lord said:

One who is not averse to illumination, hard work or delusion when they are present, nor desires them when they are absent...

23

Who is detached, undisturbed by the different qualities, firm in the knowledge that the qualities alone are active...

24

Who is centered on the self, equal to happiness or distress,
to earth, stone, or gold, to the desirable or the undesirable,
to praise or blame…

25

Who is unaffected by honor or dishonor, neutral among
friends and enemies, who gives up all selfish endeavours—
such a person, Arjuna, is said to have transcended the qualities of nature.

A WANDERING TEACHER ONCE VISITED the court of a king. The
king inquired of him, 'How is the soul bound to this world?'
In answer the wanderer tightly embraced a pillar of the king's
palace while calling, 'Release me!' In this way the soul is bound
to this world both by attachment and aversion to nature. Krishna's advice is to be neutral toward all three qualities, neither
attached nor detached, accepting goodness, passion and darkness as belonging to the tapestry of life. Goodness enlightens
and brings peace, passion encourages work and creativity, darkness brings rest and forgetfulness. All have their place in the
passage of life. We are advised neither to desire nor abhor them,
but to accept all that the Lord gives and so be free.

FOUNDATION OF ALL

26

One who serves me with unfailing devotion rises above these qualities of material nature and achieves the level of Brahman.

27

I am the basis of the immortal and imperishable Brahman, the abode of everlasting truth and ultimate happiness.

KRISHNA ANSWERS ARJUNA'S FINAL question, 'How does one transcend the qualities of nature?' He has already explained that a person who is neutral toward the qualities transcends them. But how, when our nature is to be attached, do we achieve neutrality? The answer is to give our attachment to the eternal Lord and thus become neutral toward his creation. This means that instead of serving material nature we endeavor to serve Krishna in *bhakti yoga* and so become free. This surrender brings the soul to the level of *Brahman*, above the qualities of nature. On this spiritual level of *Brahman* the soul shares the same spiritual nature as the Lord, and the eternal exchange of love between the soul and God awakens, full of truth and happiness.

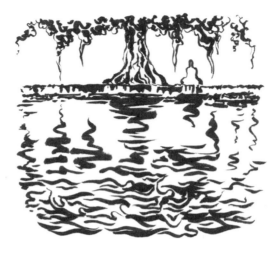

15

THE SUPREME PERSON

The World Tree extends in all directions
to envelop all struggling souls. Souls who
free themselves from this tree seek the Supreme Person
who dwells in the hearts of all. They enter
the realm of everlasting light.

THE WORLD TREE

1

The Blessed Lord said:

It is said there is an eternal banyan tree with roots above and branches below, whose leaves are the sacred hymns. One who knows this tree understands the sacred wisdom.

2

The tree's branches extend upward and downward, nourished by the qualities of nature, and their shoots are the pleasures of the senses. Its roots also go downward, bound to the actions of the human world.

3

The form of this tree is not visible to those in this world. They cannot see where it ends, where it begins, or where its foundation is. Cut down this deep-rooted tree with the weapon of detachment.

4

Thereafter, seek the place from which one never returns, and there surrender to the original Supreme Person from whom all this has extended since time immemorial.

THE COMPLEX WEB OF THE MATERIAL WORLD is symbolised by the World Tree. The tree is upside down because it is rooted in the highest reality and extends down into the world of shadows. It is a reflection of the real tree of the spiritual world, like the illusory tree reflected upside down in the water along the bank of a river.

Leaves give shade; the leaves of this tree are the sacred writings that give relief to those who shelter beneath them. A banyan tree grows secondary roots that hang from its branches; the World Tree has secondary roots bound to human actions. Our actions while living as humans on earth create karmic reactions that shape our future lifetimes in other parts of the tree. These karmic roots are deep and bind us to further existence within the tree.

So long as we are attached to the World Tree we will continue to wander from branch to branch, not knowing where it begins or ends. But if we give up our attachment, following Krishna's repeated advice throughout the *Gita*—neither clinging to the tree nor pushing it away—it will cease to bind us and we will be able to cut down its illusory form.

THE LUMINOUS WORLD

5

That everlasting place is reached by the wise who are free from pride, illusion and false attachments, ever devoted to the spirit, finished with material desires, and freed from the dualities of happiness and distress.

6

That place is not lit by the sun, or moon or fire. Those who go there never return—that is my supreme abode.

THE ETERNAL WORLD IS SELF-LUMINOUS and has no need of light. In contrast this world is dark. When our sun sets this world reverts to shadows. In the deep hollows of space where the light of the sun never reaches, permanent darkness reigns.

Therefore this world is a place of darkness. Yet we are creatures of the sun, naturally attracted to light. Similarly, though in this world of death where all beings must die, we are creatures of life who resist the very idea of death. These are some of the clues pointing to another level of reality to which we belong. That reality is described by Krishna as a place whose natural state is light.

Krishna's home is called Goloka Vrindavan. In sacred Hindu literature it is desribed as a place made of spirit where everything is full of bliss. In a forest of desire trees Krishna herds cows and plays games full of laughter and love with his friends. Krishna's form is childlike because he and his friends are ageless. Although Krishna never leaves Goloka, he is spread everywhere by his dazzling effulgence, which pervades and supports all beings and all worlds.

THE SOUL'S JOURNEY THROUGH THE WORLD

7

The souls in this world are eternal particles of myself, struggling to carry the material mind and senses.

8

Leaving one body and entering another, they carry the mind and senses with them as the wind carries the fragrance of a flower.

9

Thus ruling the ears, eyes, tongue, nose and sense of touch, grouped about the mind, the soul enjoys the pleasures of this world.

10

Those who are deluded do not understand how a soul enjoys life in the body under the spell of nature and then departs— but with the eye of knowledge this can be seen.

11

Those who strive on the path of yoga see the self within. Those who do not develop self-understanding, however they try, see nothing.

AS A PARTICLE OF GOD EACH OF US has a small part of his potencies. Wishing to play as gods, we enter this world and attract to ourselves an aura of material energy, made of mind and senses, that gives subtle shape to our desires. This subtle shape, when clothed in a physical body, gives the soul a material form through which it can manipulate and enjoy matter. We can understand from Krishna's description that the physical senses of a particular body are extensions of the subtle senses which the soul carries from one body to another. Similarly, those subtle senses are themselves emanations of the eternal spiritual senses of the soul.

Being only a very small fragment of God, in enjoying the world the soul comes under the spell of God's deluding energy, called *maya*. Forgetting our eternal spiritual identity, we are bewildered into accepting the covering of mind and senses as our true self.

Deep down, however, as we travel from one body to another, we retain the memory of our true selves, and with it the knowledge of our loving relationship with the Supreme Lord. This memory haunts us, and inspires us to search for perfect love in this world. As eternal beings we cannot bear the repeated experience of death, or having to part from those we love. In our pursuit of love and happiness we suffer the pains and misfortunes of this imperfect existence. Sometimes in this frustrated state we hear the voice of the Supersoul reminding us from within of our spiritual nature, or we hear from the sources of sacred wisdom, or from the mouths of realized souls. Then spiritual knowledge arises in our hearts and we awaken on the path of spiritual self-development.

THE SUPREME PERSON

12

The splendor of the sun, illuminating this world and reflected in the light of the moon and the glow of fire is mine.

13

I enter the earth, holding her in space and sustaining all creatures. I become the moon, giving flavor and nourishment to all plants.

14

I dwell in all living bodies as the fire of digestion, and with the vital airs digest all kinds of foods.

15

I am seated in everyone's heart. From me come remembrance, knowledge and forgetfulness. All sacred books lead to me, their knower and creator.

16

There are two kinds of beings in this world: the transient and the eternal. Created beings are transient; when they are united with the Supreme they are eternal.

17

Besides these is the highest person called the Supersoul, the eternal God who enters this world and maintains it.

18

I am beyond the transient and above even the eternal; therefore I am celebrated in the world and in the Vedas as that Supreme Person.

19

Those who know me without doubt as the Supreme Person know everything, and absorb themselves wholly in my service, Arjuna.

20

I have now disclosed to you this most secret teaching, sinless one. Understanding this you are enlightened and all your endeavours are made perfect.

THE VOICE OF KRISHNA DIRECTS US to worship the Supreme Lord as the One without a second—the original eternal person who is the source of all other eternal persons. He lives in everything giving life and support. How do planets float weightlessly in space, perfectly maintaining their orbits? We take such perfection for granted, but these arrangements are the work of the Supersoul who keeps all bodies on their courses. If for a moment he ceased his work we would perish.

While passing from one lifetime to another, the soul forgets the past. This forgetfulness is also a gift of God. If we did not forget, how could we continue to live? The pain of separation from those we love is mitigated by passing time to make it possible for us to undertake new ventures and discover new truths.

All is known to our subconscious selves, but such knowledge is more than we could bear in the midst of the illusions of material life. We have chosen to forget so that we can experience independence from God and learn what we must learn. That forgetfulness is God's gift. When the time comes for us to remember the truth again, the memory of ourselves and the understanding it brings are also gifts of God.

He is with us all the time, inviting us to give him our love. This is the highest teaching of the *Bhagavad Gita*. The great paradox of life is that the things that are most dear to us turn out to be the things we already have—food, water, air, sunlight, life itself, and the love of those near to us. It is only when we lose these most basic things that we appreciate how good they are.

When the light of the sun is hidden behind the clouds we long to see the sun again, and when its warm light returns to us our spirits are uplifted. Yet the sun, and every one of nature's blessings, are manifestations of Krishna. He is with us always. Our greatest blessing is his constant friendship. When we understand this we will return Krishna's love with our devotion and service in all we do. That spirit of service will make everything clear and our lives will be complete.

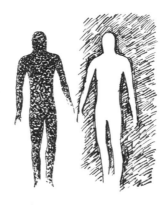

16

LIGHT AND DARK

Two kinds of beings live in this world: the divine
and the demoniac. The demoniac create misery
for themselves and others and sink into darkness.
Avoid therefore the gates to darkness – lust,
anger and greed – by heeding the sacred
books of wisdom.

DIVINE AND DEMONIAC NATURES

1–3

The Blessed Lord said:

These are the qualities that belong to those born to the divine nature: fearlessness, purification of one's existence, cultivation of spiritual knowledge, generosity, self-control, willingness to serve, study of the sacred books, austerity, simplicity, nonviolence, truthfulness, freedom from anger, renunciation, tranquility, aversion to faultfinding, compassion for all beings, freedom from craving, gentleness, modesty, steady determination, energy, forgiveness, fortitude, cleanliness, and freedom from malice and pride.

4

These belong to those born to the demoniac nature: hypocrisy, arrogance, conceit, anger, harshness and ignorance.

5

It is said that the divine nature leads to freedom and the demoniac to bondage. Do not fear, Arjuna, for you were born to the divine nature.

THE DIVINE QUALITIES of the soul can be covered by the mantle of the demoniac nature, as illustrated in the story of the gatekeepers of heaven. These two eternal servants of Vishnu chose to enter this world in the garb of demons for three lifetimes. In each life they caused terror and destruction before being slain by Vishnu and returning to be his eternal servants. Their names are Jaya and Vijaya, and their images adorn the gateposts of temples of Vishnu, recalling the soul's capacity to choose illusion. Their example teaches that those who seem demoniac are in a temporary condition and will eventually return to Krishna.

We have already learned that forgetfulness is a gift of God. If a soul desires to forget the love of God, even to the extent of wishing to kill him, God covers that soul with a veil of oblivion and gives the soul a birth that will lead to the demoniac nature. Likewise, for those who have chosen to journey toward God, birth into the divine nature leads them on that Godly journey. Most of us experience both tendencies, toward and away from God, and our higher nature must struggle with a darker side. Krishna urges us to choose goodness and light.

In the space between lives, a soul chooses to reenter the world. The soul is attracted to a particular womb to develop a body and mind that express that soul's desires through a particular combination of the qualities of nature. Once born we are bound to follow the nature we have chosen, but we can still choose our future destination according to how we live this present life. Each moment offers us a choice of whom we wish to be.

THE DARK SIDE

6

Two kinds of beings are created in this world: the divine and the demoniac. The divine have been described at length— now hear about the demoniac.

7

The demoniac do not know what is to be done and what is not to be done. No purity, good conduct or truth are found in them.

8

They say this world has no meaning, no cause and no God; that it arises from nothing more than the passionate combination of male and female.

9

Holding these misguided views and lost to themselves, they become enemies of the world, flourishing through harmful and destructive works.

10

Ruled by insatiable lust, filled with hypocrisy and pride, they are deluded by false ideas and sworn to impure work.

11

Convinced that nothing is higher than the gratification of their desires, they are beset with immeasurable fears ending only with death.

12

Bound by an endless web of desires, absorbed in lust and anger, they amass wealth by dishonest means for the satisfaction of their ambitions.

THE DEMONIAC NATURE appears from these verses to be a disease of the soul—a delusional state that is based on a denial of all that is good. We have learned from Krishna that the quality of darkness can overwhelm the other two qualities of nature in this world. It is clear that a soul caught up in the demoniac nature is ruled by this force of darkness and destruction.

A symptom of the state of darkness is surrender to sensual pleasures. Pleasure comes of its own accord as part of a balanced life. But when the mind becomes obsessed with the pursuit of pleasure and enslaved by it, pleasure turns to pain and obscures the spirit. A person in this condition falls under the power of the senses into a downward spiral leading to madness and fear, as was vividly described in the second chapter. This experience becomes a nightmare from which there is no escape, except by the grace of God.

The powers of darkness are at work wherever the few profit from the misfortune of the many. Today the planet's soil, air and water are being poisoned by the activities of a minority of people who have grown powerful under the influence of darkness. They are careless of the welfare of the planet and its inhabitants. The ambitions of just a few such people are causing havoc for everyone else.

MIND OF DARKNESS

13

'I have gained this much today toward achieving my ambitions. This wealth is mine, and more will be mine tomorrow.

14

'I have destroyed my enemy and I will destroy others too. I am in control, I enjoy as I please, I am successful, powerful and happy.

15

'I am wealthy and aristocratic. No one is my equal. I shall make sacrifice, give in charity and celebrate.' Deluded by ignorance, the mind of darkness thinks like this.

16

Distracted by countless worries, bound by a network of illusions and addicted to sense enjoyment, the demoniac fall into the depths of darkness.

17

Conceited and obstinate, proud and intoxicated with their wealth, they make a show of religion without caring for its true form or meaning.

18

Overcome by ego, power, arrogance, lust and anger, these envious people hate me in their own bodies and in others.

19

Birth after birth, I throw these cruel, hateful and degraded people into the wombs of the demoniac.

20

Born repeatedly among the demoniac and not reaching me, these deluded ones sink ever downward.

THESE VERSES PAINT a frightening picture of the demoniac mind, which thinks nothing of killing those who get in its way. People with such minds, seeing all competitors as enemies, drag those around them into conflicts, inciting wars and massacres. The root of their disordered and destructive behavior is God-hatred and self-hatred. Their spiritual propensity for love turns to hatred toward God, toward others and toward themselves.

Two questions need to be answered here. How can a soul, loving by nature, develop such a hateful condition? And how can a compassionate God throw the deluded soul repeatedly into such darkness? If we consider our experience of darkness we will get some idea. When we turn from the sun we see our shadow, for in this world all that is required for darkness to be present is the absence of light. Similarly, when the doors to the soul are firmly closed, an illusory form of darkness appears. This shadow form resembles the self, but has no real substance. We have heard in the fourteenth chapter that the quality of darkness is part of the nature of this world of matter. Its basic characteristic is ignorance, an absence of understanding. A person covered by darkness has no conception of right and wrong, and no regard for the guidance of scripture.

The scriptures say that God is neutral toward all beings, and responds to their desires without prejudice. If a soul wishes to forget God utterly, God puts that soul in the state of darkness so the soul will never have to perceive him. However, Krishna does not forget that soul, and by his grace the soul may eventually be woken from oblivion. We are told that Krishna comes to slay those who are completely lost, putting an end to their nightmare. The gates that open on darkness and close on the soul can be reopened. These gates are described in the following verses.

DOORS TO DARKNESS

21

Three gates of self-destruction lead to this place of darkness: lust, anger, and greed. Therefore give up these three.

22

A person who escapes these three gates of darkness works for self-improvement and then reaches the supreme destination.

23
One who behaves whimsically, rejecting the teachings of the
scriptures, is unable to achieve perfection, happiness or the
highest goal.

24
Therefore be guided in how to live and what to avoid by
learning from sacred books, and live in this world by their
teachings.

HAVING EXPLAINED THE PERILS of the demoniac nature, Krishna
urges us at all costs to avoid the gates that lead to it. Lust, greed,
and anger are everywhere evident in a world dominated by the
quality of passion; but they are to be neither condemned nor
encouraged. Krishna's advice has already been given at the end
of the fourteenth chapter, that one should be neutral toward
them, for aversion is another side of attachment. However, to
cultivate the urges of lust, greed and anger is to open the gates
to darkness.

We live in times when the dangers of these gates are not
generally understood. The human urges of lust, greed and anger
are encouraged by commercial interests that seek to profit from
the darker side of human nature. The proliferation of loveless
sex, intoxication, harmful technology and weapons of destruction is part of the result. A more profound effect of opening
these doors to darkness is that the doors of the soul are closed.
In a world of hardship this is the greatest cruelty, for it takes
from people their vision and hope. The greatest love one can
show others is to help them reawaken their divine nature, bring-
ing to their lives a vision of truth, hope and joy.

Light and Dark

The teachings of all the world's religions agree that lust, greed and anger must be overcome if we wish to have peace. To help us understand this spiritual psychology, for our individual welfare and the future welfare of human society, Krishna describes in detail the symptoms of the qualities of nature in the remaining two chapters.

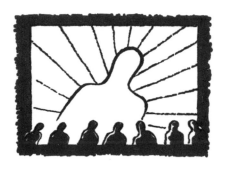

17

THREE KINDS OF FAITH

Faith is of three kinds: faith in the divine, faith
in the powers of this world and faith in spirits.
People each have different faiths, eat different
foods and sacrifice for different causes.
Without faith they can achieve nothing.

THREE FAITHS

1

Arjuna said:

Krishna, what of those who worship with faith but do not follow the guidance of scripture? Are they in goodness, passion or darkness?

2

The Blessed Lord said:

Souls in this world develop faith of three kinds according to their natures of goodness, passion or darkness. Now hear about these.

3

One's faith expresses one's own nature. A person is made of faith and faith makes a person.

4

Those in goodness worship the gods; those in passion worship demons and powerful beings; those in darkness worship ghosts and the spirits of the departed.

5–6

Apart from these are those who, driven by lust and attachment, full of hypocrisy and pride, undergo harsh penances not recommended in the scriptures. They senselessly torture their bodies as well as me within them. Their intentions are demoniac.

THROUGH THE POWER OF FAITH, people see what they believe, rather than believe what they see. The nature a person is born with, influenced by subsequent experiences, leads to that person's individual faith. Persuasion and argument cannot change a person's faith unless that person is willing to change. Faith changes and develops through experience, prayer and association with people of faith.

Three classes of faithful person are recognized by Krishna. As already assured in the seventh chapter, Krishna helps all these, strengthening their faith and giving them the results they aspire for. But those who torture their bodies have faith in no one, and consequently gain nothing except darkness.

This section of the *Bhagavad Gita* classifies people's behavior and inclinations according to the different qualities of nature. These are archetypes rather than distinct groups of people. Each of us has a nature made up of all three qualities. These classifications are guidance to help us understand our nature and the consequences of our actions, and to make good choices in life.

THREE FOODS

7

People are attracted to three kinds of food, sacrifice, penance and giving. Now hear their classifications.

8

Foods that are tasty, wholesome and satisfying, that give long life, vitality, strength, health, happiness and satisfaction, are liked by those in goodness.

9

Foods that are excessively bitter, sour, salty, hot, acidic or dry, causing discomfort, misery, and disease, are liked by those in passion.

10

Foods not freshly cooked, tasteless, decomposed or stale,
consisting of leftovers and impure things, are liked by those
in darkness.

OUR CHOICE OF FOOD AFFECTS OUR STATE of health in body, mind
and spirit. The system of Ayurvedic medicine recommends the
appropriate food for the health of the body according to our
physical type. For peace of mind and good karma one should
eat vegetarian foods, causing less violence and taking less of the
planet's resources. And for spiritual well-being, food cooked
with love and devotion is beneficial, since consciousness goes
into cooking. Best of all is food offered to Krishna.

THREE KINDS OF SACRIFICE

11

Sacrifice made according to scripture as a matter of duty,
with no desire for reward, is in goodness.

12

Sacrifice made for the sake of a reward or out of pride, is in
passion.

13

Sacrifice that is faithless, with no regard for scripture, prayers,
or the religious, in which no food is distributed, is in darkness.

THE INTENTION OF THE WORSHIPER matters more than the
outward form of a sacrifice or a religious ritual. Most worship
in human society is performed for the sake of material reward

or security. Since God is the father of all, it is natural to ask him for material benefits, such as praying for daily bread. Religion certainly brings prosperity and many blessings, but the goal of religion is to bring union with God. This comes only to those who sacrifice without attachment, out of duty or love.

THREE PENANCES

14

Penance of the body is to serve God, the devout, the teacher and superiors, and to be clean, simple, chaste and nonviolent.

15

Penance of the voice is to speak what is truthful, pleasing, edifying and gentle, and to recite the scriptures.

16

Penance of the mind is peacefulness, simplicity, silence, self-control and purity of heart.

17

This threefold penance, performed with great faith by those devoted to the Supreme and not desiring material rewards, is called penance in goodness.

18

Penance done for the sake of show, to earn respect, honor, and worship, that is unsteady and does not last, is in passion.

19

That misguided penance that tortures the self, seeking to harm others, is in darkness.

HUMAN LIFE is meant for penance. The penances recommended here, of body, words and mind, bring illumination and happiness. A life without penance, with no sacrifice for a higher cause, will not bring satisfaction. Extreme penance that hurts the body or mind is not recommended for any purpose.

THREE KINDS OF CHARITY

20

Charity given selflessly to a worthy person at the right time and place is in goodness.

21

Charity given grudgingly to gain some advantage is in passion.

22

Charity given to unworthy people, at an improper place and time, without care or respect, is in darkness.

LIFE BRINGS MANY OPPORTUNITIES to give to those who need help. Such chances bestow benefit upon the giver as well as the receiver. Therefore those who ask for help are a blessing to the rest of us. But as with sacrifice and penance, the motivation is important. If we give selflessly our love will increase. And if we give selflessly, while remembering the Supreme, we will be released from material life. The greatest gift we can give to others is knowledge of the self and of God, for that is the key to end all suffering.

OM TAT SAT

23

Om Tat Sat—these three words represent Absolute Truth. They were used to consecrate priests, scriptures and sacrifices.

24

Those who follow the Vedas therefore always begin their sacrifice, penance and charity by chanting Om.

25

Those who seek liberation, not desiring personal reward, make sacrifice, penance or charity while chanting Tat.

26

To represent truth and goodness, and on any auspicious occasion, chant Sat.

27

Sat denotes dedication to sacrifice, penance and charity and anything done with such intentions.

28

Sacrifice, penance or charity practiced without faith are called asat, and are of no consequence in this life or the next.

THE MANTRA OM TAT SAT INVOKES the presence of the Supreme Lord at all times and places. By chanting this mantra, or the Hare Krishna mantra, or any transcendental mantra containing the names of God, all of life can be sanctified.

Faith of some kind, even if it is not transcendental faith, is needed. Faith requires an openness to trusting others and looking for the good in them. At this point in the *Gita*, having heard how to discriminate between the apparent good and bad in this world, we can do well to remember that it is easy to see the faults in others, but it takes some effort to find their good qualities. The faults we see elsewhere reflect our own faults, for it is easier to see them in others than to admit them in ourselves. However, the faults we see are not to be hated. They are to be recognized and learned from.

On the spiritual path we develop different ways of seeing the world. The beginner sees God in the place of worship, in the standard religious practices, and in the scriptures. Next we perceive the presence of God more widely: in the Supreme Lord, in his devotees, in the innocent, and in those who hate God. One who sees these four relates differently to each: surrendering to God; serving his devotees; befriending the innocent; and avoiding the hateful. A further level of perception may be given by God's grace: to see God present everywhere and all beings as his servants. A person with this vision makes no distinction between the divine and the demoniac, seeing past all external coverings to recognize the soul within and the Supersoul in all.

These three ways of spiritual vision of the world each occur naturally in the life of a devotee of God. Beginning with faithful worship of the Lord and learning from others who have faith, we can discover truth and goodness even where it is hard to see. In this way we will find God in all the world and be happy.

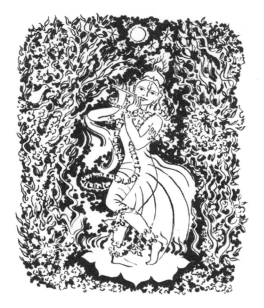

18

THE FINAL MESSAGE

All occupations, however imperfect, find
perfection in the service of God. 'Abandon all
paths and just remember me,' concludes Krishna,
'I will release you from fear.'

RENOUNCING THE RESULTS OF WORK

1
Arjuna said:
Dear Krishna, I want to understand the nature of
detachment and renunciation.

2
The Blessed Lord said:
Renunciation is giving up work that is selfish, and detach-
ment is giving up the results of work. So say the learned.

3
Some consider all work should be given up as flawed,
whereas others say works of sacrifice, charity and penance
should never be given up.

4
Listen to my conclusion about detachment, which is said to
be of three kinds.

5
Works of sacrifice, charity and penance should never be
given up, for they purify even the wise.

6
But such work should be done without wishing to enjoy the
results. This is my firm opinion.

7
Religious obligations should not be given up. Such misguided
renunciation is said to be in darkness.

8
To give up work as troublesome, so as to avoid discomfort,
brings no merit and is renunciation in passion.

9

To work as a matter of duty, without attachment for results, is renunciation in goodness.

10

The wise renouncer of the world, full of goodness and free of doubts, neither avoids unpleasant work, nor seeks pleasant work.

11

A soul living in this world cannot entirely give up work; but one who gives up the results of work is truly renounced.

12

Those who desire to enjoy the results of their actions will receive those results after death—pleasant, unpleasant and mixed. Not so the one who is detached.

No one likes to be forced to work. But in this world we cannot renounce work, for we must work to survive. Work, however, is about far more than simple survival or earning material wealth. From the standpoint of the *Gita* we learn that work offers the path to freedom and spiritual fulfillment. Even those whose work is not of their own choosing can find satisfaction by working in a spirit of detachment.

It is important to understand the difference between immediate and long-term benefit. Pleasant work may bring immediate satisfaction, but work as a sacrifice brings long-term happiness. In any case, the one who works without attachment for reward receives the greatest benefit of work, namely spiritual freedom. The way to cultivate this spirit of detachment is to remember that the self, as spirit separate from the body and mind, is not the direct cause of work. This is made clear by Krishna in the following verses.

FIVE CAUSES OF ACTION

13

Learn from me the five causes for the success of any action, as they are taught in scripture.

14

The place of action, the actor, the senses, the endeavour, and ultimately the Divine:

15

These five are the causes of whatever is done, right or wrong, with body, words or mind.

16

One who sees only the self as actor sees imperfectly and without intelligence.

17

Even one who slays all these people—if acting without ego and with clear intelligence—slays no one and is not bound.

WE MAY THINK WE ARE ALONE in doing all our work, but there are five causes of action described here. The first cause is our desire. Although we supply the desire, the fulfilment of our desire comes only with the help of the other four causes: the place of action, namely the body; the senses and organs of the body that supply the endeavour; the vital energies that flow within the body; and ultimately the divine sanction of the Supersoul.

We cannot understand how our heart beats or how our digestion functions. Nor do we know how, when we wish to learn a new skill, we are able to do so. Ultimately all this is made possible by the Supersoul who lives within us. The Supersoul is the source of instinct, the inner impulse to act in ways that have not been externally taught.

If we remain always conscious of the Supersoul, without whom we can do nothing, all our work will assume a divine dimension inspired from within. Such work is not whimsical; it is directed by the Supersoul. Work in such a spirit cannot bind us. Even Arjuna, fighting as a soldier according to his nature and his duty, remains free from karma by working in this spirit.

THREE KINDS OF KNOWLEDGE

18

Knowledge, the objects of knowledge, and the knower are the three impulses to action. The senses, the work and the actor are the three ingredients of action.

19

Now I will explain to you the three kinds of knowledge, work and actor, according to the science of the three qualities of nature.

20

Knowledge that perceives in all beings one imperishable nature, one in many, is in goodness.

21

Knowledge that perceives in all beings different natures, each separate from the other, is in passion.

22

Knowledge which is attached to one kind of work as if it were all, which is meagre and not founded on any truth, is said to be in darkness.

THOSE WHO ARE ENLIGHTENED by goodness see the underlying unity of all beings because of their shared inner nature. They honor the same spirit present in animals and plants as in humans. Those influenced by passion pay more attention to outer differences and encourage party spirit and rivalry. Darkness blinds us to anything except outer form and is insensitive to the varieties of nature that distinguish one being from another.

THREE KINDS OF WORK AND THREE ACTORS

23

Work done in the course of duty, without like or dislike, with no desire to enjoy a result, is said to be in goodness.

24

Work done egotistically to satisfy selfish desires and with great effort, is said to be in passion.

25

Work done in illusion, whimsically, without care for consequences, loss or pain, is said to be in darkness.

26

The actor without selfish attachment or ego, steadfast and determined, unwavering in success or failure, is said to be in goodness.

27

The actor full of desire and motivated by results, who is greedy, aggressive and impure, easily moved to elation or depression is said to be in passion.

28

The actor who is undisciplined, vain, obstinate, deceitful, rude, lazy, morose and procrastinating is said to be in darkness.

ONE INFLUENCED BY GOODNESS is not led by the superficial likes and dislikes of the mind and likes to do what is worth doing as a matter of duty. It is better to see an action in terms of its consequences, to know clearly why it should be done, than to be ruled by the whims of the mind.

THREE KINDS OF UNDERSTANDING AND WILL

29

Now hear from me in detail of the different kinds of understanding and will, according to the three qualities of nature.

30

Understanding when to act or not act, what to do or avoid doing, what is harmful or safe and what binds or gives freedom, is in goodness.

31

Understanding that cannot distinguish right from wrong, or what to do from what to avoid doing, is in passion.

32

Understanding clouded by illusion, that thinks wrong to be right and sees everything backward, is in darkness.

33

The will made unfailing by yoga practice, that holds firmly the mind, senses and life energy, is in goodness.

34

The will that clings to duty, wealth and pleasure, desiring their fruits, is in passion.

35

The will of a foolish person, preoccupied with dreams, fear, grief, depression and illusion, is in darkness.

REGULAR PRACTICE OF YOGA steadies the mind and opens the heart to the inner peace of the soul. This makes a person self-sufficient and able to live without always being dependent for happiness on external stimuli for the mind or senses. In this state of mind it is easier to hear and understand the wisdom of scripture, and to have it confirmed from within by the voice of the Supersoul. Then it is possible to understand what to do or not to do, and to act with steady conviction.

THREE KINDS OF HAPPINESS

36

Now hear from me of the three kinds of happiness whose repeated enjoyment eventually brings an end to distress.

37

Happiness arising from the calm of self-understanding, that seems like poison in the beginning but turns to nectar in the end, is said to be in goodness.

38

Happiness based on the pleasures of the senses, that seems like nectar in the beginning but turns to poison in the end, is said to be in passion.

39

Happiness arising from sleep, laziness and forgetfulness, that is self-delusion from beginning to end, is said to be in darkness.

40

No being on earth or among the gods in heaven is free of the influence of the three qualities of goodness, passion or darkness.

WE NEED TO BE HAPPY, but the happiness of this world cannot satisfy the soul. Worldly happiness is like a drop of water in the desert—enough to make us want more but not enough to satisfy. This world is not a happy place because all who are born must experience disease, old age, and finally death. Yet in the midst of pain the heart continues to hope for happiness because our spirit is *ananda,* joyful.

The best kind of happiness, therefore, is the kind that may begin with hardship, but grows steadily with time. This is the happiness of goodness. If we follow the principles of the *Bhagavad Gita* we can taste this happiness.

The happiness of passion ends in disappointment because it is based on the temporary pleasures of the senses. When the body is young it is attractive and everyone wants to see and touch it; as the body ages it loses its appeal; in old age we mourn the lost pleasures of youth. Although we will be offered the chance to be reborn and taste again those pleasures, we will also have to experience again their loss and the pain of old age. This disappointment will be repeated until we learn to look within, and to Krishna, for happiness.

The rewards of passion soon pall. If the soul will not turn to Krishna, disillusion turns the soul toward darkness and forgetfulness, and to the oblivion of sleep and intoxication. However, the possibility of awakening to the spiritual joy of the soul is always present by the grace of Krishna. The joy of the spirit brings happiness beyond all three kinds of material happiness.

This section completes Krishna's teachings on the three qualities of nature. Finally Krishna urges us to follow our duties in life, summarized in the following verses. By following these each of us can use our natural good qualities to gradually be elevated, regardless of our present position.

THE FOUR OCCUPATIONS

41

The duties of intellectuals, leaders, merchants and workers are classed according to their natural qualities.

42

Peacefulness, self-control, penance, purity, forgiveness, honesty, knowledge, wisdom and faith in God—these are the natural duties of intellectuals.

43

Courage, strength, determination, resourcefulness, facing the enemy, generosity and command are the natural duties of leaders.

44

Farming, cow protection and trade are the natural duties of merchants, and service is the natural duty of the workers.

45

By following your natural duty you can achieve perfection. Hear from me how.

46

By worshiping with your work the One from whom all beings emanate and by whom all is pervaded, you can achieve perfection.

47

The occupation given to you, though imperfect, is better than another's, even perfectly done. Doing your natural duty never brings sin.

48

Do not give up your natural work, even if it is faulty, for all undertakings have some fault, as fire is covered by smoke.

THE HEART OF KRISHNA'S MESSAGE, given in the tenth chapter, is to absorb ourselves fully in his service, remembering him constantly. But how will an ordinary person accomplish this precious instruction? Here, almost at the end of his teaching, Krishna advises how, by carrying out the work nature has assigned to us, and worshiping the Lord with that work, even though that work may be imperfect we can achieve perfection.

The four occupations Krishna describes here are the four classes of the Vedic society: *brahmana, kshatriya, vaishya, sudra.* These correspond to natural archetypes found in all human societies and are a general guide for applying the principle of sacred work. The principle is to know our natural inclination, cultivate the good qualities associated with it, and work accordingly while thinking of God.

All work is bound to have shortcomings, particularly in today's disordered world. There are times when our principles must be compromised for the sake of our work, or when our work is compromised by the constraints of the world. Krishna recognizes this and still encourages us. In Arjuna's case, his work is to protect others. Krishna urges him on, even though the fight is abhorrent to him and beset with moral dilemmas. We each have to face tests and difficult choices. If we follow the principles taught by Krishna we will find that we have his support and protection in everything that we do.

SPIRITUAL JOY

49

One who is intellectually detached, self-controlled, and without desires can by practice of renunciation attain perfect freedom from karma.

50

Arjuna, learn from me briefly how by achieving this perfection you also attain Brahman, the stage of highest knowledge.

51

With clear intelligence and controlled mind, disregarding outside sensations such as sound, putting aside likes and dislikes,

52-53

Living in seclusion, eating little, controlling thought, word and deed, absorbed always in meditation, cultivating detachment, abandoning ego, power, pride, lust, anger, possessions, with no sense of ownership and being peaceful—in this way you achieve Brahman.

54

One absorbed in Brahman is full of spiritual joy and no longer laments or desires. Such a person, being equal toward all beings, attains pure devotion for me.

THESE VERSES RETURN US to the theme of the sixth chapter by describing the path of complete renunciation of the world. They are spoken in response to Arjuna's question about renunciation at the beginning of this chapter.

A small number of men and women in all societies are called away from the world to a life of penance, prayer and contemplation. Their path leads them to the *Brahman* consciousness, where they experience everything as spirit and enjoy spiritual rapture free from all anxieties.

Those who remain serving Krishna in the world and those who contemplate *Brahman* in solitude both arrive ultimately at the same place: pure devotion for Krishna. This perfect stage of self-surrender marks the entrance to eternal life.

So we are brought to the final passage of verses, which are unsurpassed among the sacred books of the world. They give us the sublime conclusion to Krishna's teachings in the *Bhagavad Gita*.

PERFECT DEVOTION

55

Through devotion you will know all about me, and in truth who I am. Once you know me truly, you can enter my abode.

56

Though working in all kinds of ways under my protection, my devotee reaches the imperishable abode by my grace.

57

Mentally surrender all your work to me, making me the goal of your life. Be absorbed on the path of devotion, always conscious of me.

58

Be conscious of me and by my grace you will overcome all difficulties. But if through ego you do not hear me, you will be lost.

59

If out of ego you decide not to fight, your resolve will be in vain, for your nature will make you fight.

60

Bound by your natural inclination you will be forced to do the very thing that in your delusion you resist.

61

The Lord dwells in the hearts of all beings, making them wander under the spell of illusion as if seated on a machine of maya.

62

Surrender to him utterly, Arjuna. By his grace you will gain ultimate peace and reach the eternal abode.

63

Thus I have told you this most secret of all secret knowledge.
Reflect on this fully, then do as you wish.

KRISHNA TAKES RESPONSIBILITY for all our wanderings. Even if
we wish to act against our nature, still we cannot. Therefore
he urges us to resign ourselves to him. However, he leaves us
a final choice. He will not force us to love him—how can he?
The choice is ours, and that precious freedom lies at the heart
of the *Gita* and the paradox of life. Though we are governed by
our natures, we are also creatures of free will. This freedom is
honored by the Lord at the cost of everything.

We imagine that we have many choices in life. But in truth
our choice is simple: to serve Krishna with love and understanding, or to be ruled by Krishna's material nature. Either way we
are servants. We are bound to serve because, though we are
eternal spiritual beings, we are small, dominated by the engulf-
ing ocean of Krishna's divine energies. These energies are called
maya and can be experienced in two ways. *Maya* can be experienced as Krishna's illusory material nature, which causes us to
forget and carries us through the revolving cycle of birth and
death. Or *maya* can be experienced as the embrace of Krishna's
spiritual nature, called *yogamaya*, the loving energy that brings
us to him. Our choice is simple: the illusion of forgetfulness, or
the embrace of Krishna's love. Within Krishna's existence the
individuality of the lover and beloved unfolds in an eternal spiritual exchange of love.

Now everything has been said, and Krishna has only to add
his closing words of love and reassurance.

The Final Message

FINAL MESSAGE OF LOVE

64

Hear once more my final message, the greatest secret of all, spoken for your benefit because you are my dearly beloved.

65

Think of me always, become my devotee, worship me and bow down to me. Thus surely you will come to me. I promise you this because you are my dear friend.

66

Abandon all kinds of religion and surrender to me alone. I will free you from all sinful reactions. Do not fear.

THE WORDS KRISHNA SPOKE at the end of the ninth chapter are here repeated: 'Think of me always.' Only this time he repeats these words as a promise of friendship.

This constant remembrance of Krishna is called Krishna consciousness. It means to live our life in such a way as to remember always the beautiful cowherd boy Krishna. Surrounded by his friends, he plays his flute and dances with his lovers in the everlasting forests of Vrindavan.

Krishna is our friend who loves us and will save us from anything. We have only to turn to him, accept his love and freely give our love in response. It is the easiest and yet the hardest thing to do: accept another's love and give our love in return.

At last it comes down to this. When all has been said in all the teachings of all the religions of the world, only two things remain: the fear of God and the love of God. Krishna consciousness is to bring us from fear to love. Choose love and all fear is gone. This is Krishna's final message.

KRISHNA'S BLESSING

67

This final secret must not be spoken to one who is not austere, not a devotee, does not wish to listen, or speaks ill of me.

68

One who teaches this supreme secret to my devotees offers me the greatest love, and without doubt comes to me.

69

No one is dearer to me than such a person, nor on earth will there ever be one more dear.

70

I declare that whoever studies this sacred dialogue of ours worships me with the intellect.

71

And whoever hears and listens with faith and open heart is liberated and reaches the blessed realms of the virtuous.

72

Dear Arjuna, have you heard with attentive mind? Are your ignorance and confusion now dispelled?

KRISHNA HAS ALREADY SAID that Arjuna should make his own choice. Now he encourages all those who in the future will study his words to do the same. Reflect deeply on this dialogue, he says, consider it from all angles, and then reach your own conclusion. The *Bhagavad Gita* is not a book of doctrine that must be accepted without question. It is to be studied and reflected upon. If we choose to put faith in Krishna, and apply his instructions in our lives, we will see for ourselves the results of heeding his words of love.

In case we should think that the love spoken of is exclusively between ourselves and Krishna, we are reminded here that all of us are bound together in this ocean of love. The perfect expression of our loving nature is to share the awareness of Krishna's love with all his separated parts who live in this world, and who forget him. This will fulfil our natural desire to love others and open us to receive their love in return.

My guru Srila Prabhupada did just this. He chose to share his love for Krishna by travelling and preaching throughout the world, and by writing many books about Krishna. He wrote, 'If we learn how to love Krishna, then it is very easy to immediately and simultaneously love every living being.'

CONCLUDING WORDS

73

Arjuna said:

My illusion is destroyed and my memory restored by your grace, Krishna. Free from doubt, I stand ready to follow your instructions.

74

Sanjaya said:

Thus I have heard this wonderful dialogue between Krishna and the great-souled Arjuna. It makes my hair stand on end.

75

By the grace of my guru, Vyasa, I have heard these supreme secrets of yoga directly from the Lord of yoga, Krishna.

76

O King, as I remember over and over these sublime and sacred words between Krishna and Arjuna, I feel joy again and again.

77

As I remember time after time Krishna's wonderful form, amazement and joy fill my heart more and more.

78

Where there is Krishna, Lord of Yoga, and the archer Arjuna, there will surely be fortune, victory, happiness and morality.

BY THE GRACE OF HIS GURU, Sanjaya heard Krishna's words. His guru was Vyasa, the author of the *Mahabharata* and the *Bhagavad Gita*. A guru is one who points the way to Krishna. It is said that without the grace of such a soul who has seen the truth, no one can find their way home.

One who chooses to surrender to Krishna is advised to search for a spiritual teacher who is a devotee of Krishna, and to practice *bhakti* yoga, devotional service, under the teacher's guidance. This act of submission opens the door of the heart to receive the blessings of the Lord. If you are unable to find such a teacher, Krishna himself will help you from within.

You have only to chant Krishna's names to fulfil all the teachings of the *Bhagavad Gita*.

Hare Krishna
Hare Krishna
Krishna Krishna
Hare Hare

Hare Rama
Hare Rama
Rama Rama
Hare Hare

Bhagavad Gita
TOPICS IN THE *BHAGAVAD GITA*

PART 1: THE SOUL IN THE WORLD

1 Arjuna's Dilemma
Prologue
The Field of Battle
Surveying the Armies
The Prospect of Disaster

2 Understanding the Soul
Arjuna's Sorrow
Submission before Krishna
The Self is Different from the Body
Tolerate the Impermanent
The Eternal Self
Do not Lament
The Honorable Warrior
Path of Freedom
Beyond the Rewards of Paradise
The Art of All Work
Leaving the Forest
The Undisturbed One
The Power of the Senses
Freedom in Self-Control
Peace in the Night

3 Karmayoga—Work and Desire
The Need to Act
The Wheel of Sacrifice
Work With Detachment
The Welfare of All
Do Not Unsettle the Ignorant
Choose to Be Free
Walk the Path Given to You
The Enemy Within

4 Transcendental Wisdom
Descent of Wisdom

Krishna's Mission
Freedom from Fear and Anger
How Karma Works
Ways of Sacrifice
Gift of Knowledge

5 Life of Freedom
Freedom Through Work
Enlightenment
Seeing with Equal Vision
The Sources of Misery
Liberation

6 Mystic Yoga
Giving Up Selfish Motivation
Make the Mind Your Friend
Happiness of the Yogi
Seeing God in All Beings
The Restless Mind
There is No Spiritual Failure

PART 2: THE MYSTERY OF GOD

7 God and His Energies
Rare Knowledge
God's Energies
God is Everywhere
Seekers of Truth
Many Faiths
God is Hidden

8 Attaining the Supreme
Ingredients of Life
How to Die
The World of Samsara
The Eternal World
Reaching the Supreme

Bhagavad Gita

9 *Most Confidential Knowledge*
Hear My Secret
Krishna is Within and Beyond Everything
Great Souls Worship Krishna
Krishna is All
Fruit of Devotion
Give Everything to Krishna
A Devotee Never Perishes

10 *The Infinity of God*
Krishna's Supreme Nature
Heart of the *Bhagavad Gita*
Arjuna's Praise
Infinite Forms of God

11 *Vision of the Universal Form*
Arjuna Desires Divine Eyes
Krishna Reveals His Universal Form
Awesome Vision
The Vision Speaks
Arjuna's Prayers
Seeing With the Eyes of Love

12 *The Way of Devotion*
Service or Meditation?
Stages On the Path
One Who Is Dear to the Lord

PART 3: THE JOURNEY

13 *Knowing the Field*
The Field of Action
The Sum of All Knowledge
The End of Knowledge
Soul and Supersoul
The Light of Wisdom

14 *The Three Qualities Of Nature*
Father of All
Nature's Three Qualities

How the Three Interact
Understanding the Three
Transcending the Three
Foundation of All

15 *The Supreme Person*
The World Tree
The Luminous World
The Soul's Journey Through the World
The Supreme Person

16 *Light and Dark*
Divine and Demoniac Natures
The Dark Side
Mind of Darkness
Doors to Darkness

17 *Three Kinds of Faith*
Three Faiths
Three Foods
Three Kinds of Sacrifice
Three Penances
Three Kinds of Charity
Om Tat Sat

18 *The Final Message*
Renouncing the Results of Work
Five Causes of Action
Three Kinds of Knowledge
Three Kinds of Work and Three Actors
Three Kinds of Understanding and Will
Three Kinds of Happiness
The Four Occupations
Spiritual Joy
Perfect Devotion
Final Message of Love
Krishna's Blessings
Concluding Words

GLOSSARY OF KEY CONCEPTS IN THE *BHAGAVAD GITA* WITH THEIR SANSKRIT TERMS

ahamkara	(*aham* 'I', *kara* 'act') illusory sense of self as being the body or the mind
akarma	inaction: action without karmic reaction (opp. karma)
apara	lower, belonging to the lower nature (opp. para)
asat	untruth; unreality (opp. *sat*)
asura	person who disobeys *dharma*, and does harm to others or to the self (opp. *sura*)
atma	self: body, mind or soul; or the Supreme Spirit (see *jivatma* and *paramatma*)
avatara	one who descends: an appearance of the divine in this world.
avidya	ignorance; lack of knowledge (opp. *vidya*)
avyakta	unmanifest, formless, inperceptible; the impersonal aspect of the Supreme; the formless uncreated state of the dormant material energy prior to or in between creations
bhagavan	Supreme Lord, possessor of opulence
bhakta	one who is devoted to the Supreme
bhakti	devotion to the Supreme
bhakti yoga	the path of devotional service to the Supreme
Brahma	the first created being, grandfather of the universe, member of the supposed Hindu trinity
brahman	the spiritual nature; the pervasive presence of the Supreme; the Supreme
brahma-nirvana	see *nirvana*
buddhi	understanding; inspired wisdom
buddhi yoga	the path of constant remembrance of the Supreme
deva	divine being; higher order of created being
dharma	universal religious principles; essential quality that unites all beings with the universe and with God
guna	one of the three primary qualities of nature: sattva guna, goodness and illumination; rajo guna, passion and creativity; tamo guna, darkness and ignorance
isvara	God, the Supreme Controller
japa	soft or silent repetition of a mantra as prayer or

	meditation, may be counted on a *japa*-mala, string of prayer beads	*para*	higher; belonging to the higher nature
jivatma	the individual soul	*paramatma*	Supreme Self, or Supersoul, who dwells within every living being
jnana	knowledge		
jnana yoga	path of knowledge of the Supreme	*parampara*	system of disciplic succession, or lineage of spiritual teaching
jnani	one who practices jnana-yoga	*prakriti*	material nature, the primordial energy of God from which the world is formed
karma	action; past actions which accrue results; hence can mean the results of past actions		
		prana	breath; vital force
karma yoga	the path of dedicating actions to the Supreme, thus gaining liberation from the results of action	*purusa*	Supreme Person; sometimes can mean the individual soul
		rajas	the material quality of passion and creativity (see guna)
karmi	one who practices karma yoga		
mantra	(man 'mind', tra 'release') spiritual sound vibration upon which to focus the mind and senses	*sadhu*	saintly person
		samadhi	mystical trance; complete absorption in the Supreme
		samsara	the seemingly endless cycle of birth, old age, disease and death
maya	'that which is not', or illusion; the creative energy of God which gives rise to illusion		
		sankhya	one of the six Vedic philosophical systems, Sankhya analyzes matter into twenty-four elements with the aim of distinguishing the soul from these twenty-four
moksha	see *mukti*		
mukti	salvation; liberation from the ties of karma and the cycle of rebirth		
nirvana	cessation of material existence; the Gita uses the term *brahma-nirvana* to indicate that after the false self is extinguished, the true self, *brahman*, remains.	*sannyasa*	complete renunciation
		sannyasi	a member of the homeless order of celibate monks
		sastra	Vedic literatures; authoritative religious text (see smriti and sruti)

sat	truth; reality	*vidya*	cultivation of knowledge; education
sattva	the material quality of goodness and illumination (see *guna*)	*visvarupa*	universal form of God, as pervading the whole universe
smriti	remembered; scriptures such as the *Puranas*, based upon discussion of the *sruti* (see *sruti*)	*yajna*	sacrifice; offering to God as form of worship
sraddha	faith in God	*yoga*	link or union, usually describes the relationship
sruti	directly heard; revealed scriptures: the Vedic hymns and *Upanishads* (see *smriti*)		between the soul and God; a spiritual discipline seeking closer union with God;
sura	godly person, who abides by *dharma*		yoga is one of the six Vedic philosophical systems
tamas	the material quality of darkness and ignorance (see *guna*)	*yogi*	one who practices yoga
		yuga	cosmic passage of time: the four yugas together
tapa	austerity and penance by exercising control of one's own senses		make a cosmic cycle lasting 4.5 million years, and a thousand such cycles make
tyaga	renunciation of the results of actions		a cosmic day. The present, fourth, yuga is *Kali Yuga*,
veda	spiritual knowledge; the ancient Sanskrit hymns directly revealed by God: *Rik Veda, Sama Veda, Yajur Veda and Atharva Veda*		a period of disorder and diminishing wisdom and life-span

INDEX

A

Abhimanyu (son of
  Subhadra), 6
Adityas, 115, 118
Action, 49, 55, 81, 100,
  123, 146, 156
  better than inaction, 30
  beyond the misery of,
    23
  bitter and sweet fruits
    of, 23
  as cause of birth and
    death, 23
  chain of, 105
  as definition of karma,
    20
  five causes of, 183
  forbidden, 46
  fruit of, 102, 129
  fundamental to self, 31
  impulses to, 184
  inaction, 46
  as inner link with God,
    xv
  made possible by the
    Lord, 36
  overcome bondage of,
    20
  produces reaction,
    20
Agni, 110
Airavata, 110
Akarma, 54
Amrita, 131
Analogies
  banyan leaves are sacred
    writings, 156

blazing fire—knowledge
  burns karma, 50
boat of knowledge, 41,
  50
controlling the wind, 68
cup of life, 93
dreamers in their
  dreams, 36
drop of water and
  ocean, 59
embryo covered by
  womb, 38
fallen yogi like
  evaporating cloud, 69
fire covered by smoke,
  38, 190
five horses reined by the
  mind, 69
fruit-bearing tree of
  karma, 102
fuel used to extinguish
  fire, 39
harvesting the fruits of
  happiness/distress, 137
intelligence as chariot
  driver, 69
irresolute mind like
  branches of tree, 20
Krishna appears like the
  sun, 44
lamp in a windless
  place, 60, 65
love of mother for child,
  99, 103
lotus leaf, 54
mind—wind;
  intelligence—boat, 26

mirror covered by dust,
  38
moths rush to flame,
  119
music carries mind of
  composer, 112-113
ocean of love, 197
ocean of misery, 41, 50
ocean of birth and
  death, 132
ocean—mind at peace;
  river—desire, 27
parents efforts hidden
  from children, 35
pearls strung on a
  thread, 75, 77
perfume, 56
poet's words carry
  thoughts, 112
rituals as small pond in
  ocean of truth, 22
ruler of the city of nine
  gates, 55
shining lamp of
  knowledge, 107
sick must follow
  restricted diet, 26
sky (self) remains pure,
  144
soul labors in the field,
  137, 139
soul like actor, 17
soul as spark of divine
  fire, 17
soul like sun, 17, 145
soul wears bodies like
  cloth, 16

205

sparks depend upon fire, 77

sun hidden behind clouds, 162

the sun lights up everything in the day, 55, 144

Krishna pervades world like sun, 96

tree reflected upside down, 156

two birds as eternal friends, 143

watering the roots of the cosmic tree, 23

waves of river hasten to ocean, 119

well-tuned radio receiver, 63

wind carries fragrance, 158

wise one's senses like tortoise, 25

worldly happiness like drop of water in desert, 188

Ananda, 188

Ananta, 110

Angels, 118

Anger, 130, 163, 164, 166, 168, 169, 171, 192

opens the gates to darkness, 170

produces illusion, 26

Arjuna, 5, 6, 7, 8, 14, 18, 24, 35, 38, 42, 51, 53, 57, 68-70, 76, 86, 89, 90, 93, 102, 105, 115, 120, 123, 153, 164, 172, 181, 184, 191, 192, 193, 196, 197, 198

accepts Krishna as teacher, 13

the archer, 198

asks for detailed knowledge, 84

becomes joyful, 123

confused, 13, 30

collapses in grief, 10

desires divine eyes, 115

devoted to Krishna, 43

as every soul, xi

enquires how to recognize the wise, 24

feels joy again and again, 198

('s) final question, 154

great-souled, 197

foresees disaster, 8

as Krishna's friend, xiv, 42

('s) mind full of fear, 122

('s) nature is to fight, 193

opens his heart to Krishna, 93

overcome with compassion, 12

('s) praise, 108, 121

('s) prayers, 121

recognizes family members, 7

shuns war, 9

surrenders to Krishna, 13

('s) vision, 117

Armies, xiv

Art of all work, v, 22, 23

Aryama, 110

Asita, 108

Astanga Yoga, 49, 59, 66

Asvatta, 112

Ashvattama, 5

Ashvins, 115, 118

Atma, 141

Atmarati, 34

Attachment, 44, 106

and aversion, 27, 37, 153

false, 157

freedom from, 24, 34

to happiness, 148

leads to desire and anger, 25

to matter, 93

relinquish all, 47

renounce, 25, 61

without worldly, 125, 182

yoga as work without, 20, 22

Ayurvedic medicine, 175

B

Banyan tree (see World Tree), 156

Battle (with mind and senses), xiv

Bhagavad Gita, 37, 51, 66, 71, 120, 145, 151, 157, 178, 192, 194, 196, 198

adopted as Hindu standard, xiii

age of, xii

based on Vedas and Upandishads, xiii

classifies behavior according to nature, 174

condensed framework, xvi, xvii

context of, 10

as dialogue of the spirit, xv

following...we can taste happiness, 188

Index

heart of (four seed verses; 10:8-11), xvi, 106, 107
the highest teaching of, 162
Krishna's invitation to join him, 97
opens cataclysmic battle, xiv
reconciles sacred and profane, 4
scripture of grace (inserted into Mahabharata), 145
for self-discovery, 22
spoken at Kurukshetra, xiv
summarizes Perennial Philosophy, xiii
summit of education, 93
synopsis of Vedic wisdom, 90
tradition, world is Mother, 10
universally accessible, xii
this version for my children, xvii
Bhagavan, possessor of opulence, 13,
Bhaktivedanta Swami (see Srila Prabhupada), xvii,
Bhakti yoga, v, 66, 71, 98, 129, 154, 198
as culmination of all yoga, 71
direct and most perfect, 128
path of personal devotion, 128
Bhima, 5,

Bhishma, 5, 7, 12, 119
Bhurishrava, son of Somadatta, 5
Bible, xi
Bliss, 57, 58, 77, 107
Body as outer dress, 13,
Brahma, 106, 117
created by Krishna, 121
('s) dawn, 88
('s) day, 87
('s) heaven, 87
Krishna is, 111
('s) planet (Brahmaloka), 88
Brahmajyoti, 107
Brahman, 47, 49, 56, 58, 59, 65, 81, 84, 86, 89, 90, 140, 141
attains, 144, 153, 191, 192
'I am the basis of', 154
emanates from Krishna, 140
Brahmana, 190
Brahma-nirvana, 59
Brahma-sutras, 138
Breath control, 48, 59
Bhrigu, 110
Brhaspati, 110
Brhat-sama hymn, 111
Buddha (Gautama), 44, 112
C
Celibacy, 86
Chanting, 98, 103, 107, 108, 118, 129, 145
great souls are always...
Krishna's glories, 97
the names of the Lord, 71, 178, 198
Om Tat Sat, 178

Charity, 178, 181
three kinds, 177
Chastity of women, 9
Chaos, 34
Chekitana, 5
Child sages (Kumaras), 106
Chitraratha, 110
Cosmic Person, 98
Cow, 56, 110, 158
protection, 190
D
Darkness (tamo guna), 149, 151, 153, 157, 163, 166, 185-188
as absence of light, 169
charity in, 177
covers knowledge, 149
dominant, 152
doors to, 169
faith in, 173
harms others, 176
illusory form of, 169
the mind of, 167
powers of, 167
qualities of, xvi, 78, 79, 148
sacrifice in, 175
Death, 75, 81, 82, 85, 86, 93, 121, 122, 139, 166, 188, 194
Krishna is all-devouring, 111
Krishna assures liberation from, 145
beyond, 97, 143
as continuous process, 87
as duality, 88
enter God's presence at, 28

god of, 110
is an illusion, 89
need not wait till...to
experience God, 28
no one wants...because
soul is eternal, 88
receive results after, 182
remembering Krishna
at, 83
all souls resist the very
idea, 158
Vedic pleasure-seekers
remain in world of, 100
world of, 157
Deerskin, 64
Delhi, xiv
Demons, 108, 110, 118,
123, 184
temporary irony of, 164,
165
those in passion
worship, 173
Demoniac, 179
mind, 168
nature, 79, 163, 164,
165, 170
as disease of the soul,
166
falls into the depths of
darkness, 168
Despondency causes
disgrace, 12
Desire, 79, 80, 106
bound by, 55
causes attachment and
then anger, 25
following...destroys
peace, 27
giving up...bestows
peace, 27
natural to the soul;

cannot be stopped, 28
obscures our perception
of God, 28
selfish...destroys self-
understanding, 29
soul's...attracts
particular womb, 165
Detachment, 13, 22, 24,
33, 121, 128, 129, 131,
139, 141, 156, 183, 193
three kinds of, 181
Determination, 19, 20, 46,
69, 130, 164, 185
impersonal path
depends upon...of
follower, 128
Devadatta, 6
Devas, 32, 33, 49, 80, 118
always long to see
Krishna's form, 124
god of death, 110
god of love, 110
god of smoke, 90
god of war, 110
worshipers of...are born
among, 100
Devala, 108
Devotee, 101, 102, 103,
107, 108, 123, 125, 129,
131, 179
'my...comes to me', 196
'is dear to me', 130
'my...is never lost to
me...', 117
never perishes, 102
Devotion (see bhakti), 43,
63, 66, 70, 80, 85, 87, 97,
98, 101, 103, 124, 126,
127, 132, 145, 153, 162,
193, 198
fruit of, 99

seed of, 107
stages of...practice, 129
plant of (devotional
service), 107
Dhristadhyumna, 4, 5
Dhritarashtra, 4, 5, 6, 8, 9,
10, 119
the sons of, 6, 12
Dhyana yoga, 71
Dishonor, 62, 130, 153
(worse than death), 19
Draupadi, the sons of, 4, 5
Dronacharya, 4, 7, 12, 119
Dhrishtaketu, 5
Drupada, 5, 6
Duryodhana, 4, 5, 7
Duty, 13, 19, 34, 42, 132,
175, 176, 182, 184, 185,
186, 187, 190
of strong to protect the
weak, 20
E
Earth, 62, 70, 77, 90, 151,
153, 157, 160, 196
Arjuna may enjoy, 19
earthly realms, 20, 88,
150, 152
dominated by passion,
150
Krishna descends to, 97
Krishna's play on, 123
souls return to...after
enjoying, 88
worshipers of power
reborn on, 100
Eating (as an expression
of love for God), 101
Ego, 35, 77, 131, 138, 139,
168, 185, 193
abandoning, 192
absence of, 139

Elephant, 56, 110
Elements (eight), 77, 85
  twenty-four, 138, 139,
Enemy, 39, 40, 63, 166,
  189
  devotee looks equally
  on friend and, 130, 153
  unsubdued mind is, 62
  within, 38
Enlightenment, xiv, 24,
  25, 33, 46, 51, 54, 57, 63,
  105, 107, 112, 150, 152,
  153, 161, 185
Equal vision, 56
Evil, 70, 151
Evolution (of bodies), 84
F
Faith, 51, 55, 65, 70, 76,
  88, 93, 107, 127, 143, 196
  three kinds of, 172
Farming, 190
Fate of the powerful, 6
Family,
  foundation of society, 9
  destruction of, 9
Fear, xvi, 13, 20, 24, 25,
  44, 45, 58, 64, 82, 101,
  105, 106, 114, 118, 119,
  120, 121, 122, 123, 124,
  130, 164, 166, 167, 180,
  187, 195, 195
  Arjuna's mind full of,
  122
  do not, 180, 195
  of God, 120, 195
Field (of action), 138,
  141, 144
  knower of, 138, 144
  nature of, 138
--
Fire,

as form of God, 99
  not used to illuminate
  Krishna's abode, 157
Fire ceremony, 49
Fire god (Agni), 110
Flower, 92
Forefathers, 118
Foods, 32, 32, 33, 63, 66,
  69, 101, 160, 162, 172,
  174, 174, 175, 175
  in darkness, 175
  three, 174
  vegetarian, 101, 175
Forest (see nirvana)
  leaving the...of delusion,
  23, 64
Forgetfulness, 26, 59, 67,
  79, 148, 149, 150, 151,
  153, 162, 188, 189,
  comes from Krishna,
  160
  is a gift from God, 161
  illusion of, 194
Forgiveness, 10, 105, 139,
  164, 189
Friendship, xii, 57, 63,
  162, 195, 195
Freedom, 48, 52, 55, 56,
  63, 106, 186
  from attachment, 24
  from bondage, 20
  from craving, 164
  divine nature leads to,
  164
  from doubt, 197
  from fear and anger, 25,
  44
  from the cycle of birth
  and death, 23
  from fear, 20
  from harm, 46

from karma, 20, 102,
  191
  human life offers, 21,
  151
  from malice and pride,
  164
  not obtained by
  avoiding work, 30
  path to, 144, 182
  sacrifice false pleasure
  for real, 27
  world moves all souls
  to, 121
  yoga of self-control
  brings, 27
G
Gambling, 47
Gandhi, Mahatma, xii
Ganges, 111
Garuda, 110
Gentle priest, 56
Ghosts, 173
Goal,
  of all sacrifice, 59
  highest, 64
  of human life, 58,
  of knowledge (Krishna),
  141
  of life, 193
  of scripture, 22
  of yoga, 66
Gold, 153
Goloka Vrindavan, 108,
  158
Goodness (sattva guna),
  150, 151, 153, 179, 184,
  185-188
  binds to happiness, 149
  charity in, 177
  enlightens and brings
  peace, 153

faith in, 173
qualities of, xvi, 77, 79, 148
sacrifice in, 175
Gospels, xiii
Govinda, 125
Grace (see Mercy)
Great sages, 105

H
Happiness, 62, 80, 81, 120, 130, 139, 157, 170, 179, 188, 189, 198
and distress are tolerated, 15, 19
achieved through unity of purpose, 21
bound by goodness, 149
doubting soul cannot find, 50
found within, 25, 58,

dependent upon each other, 32
Krishna is abode of, 154
material...limited and temporary, 39
not found by those seeking reward, 22
penance brins, 177
sacrifice bring long-term, 182
supreme, 65
three kinds of, 187
of the yogi, 64
Hare Krishna (mantra), 69, 90, 129, 178
replaces all other disciplines, 90
Hatha Yoga, 49
Healing herb, 98
Heavenly realms, 20, 99,

123, 164
Hell, 9
Himalayan mountains, 110
Hindu priests, 49
Horses (five senses), 69
Human form
affords self-development, 21
Humility, 139, 140
Huxley, Aldous, xiii

I
Iksvaku, 41
Illusion,16, 24, 35, 57, 71, 89, 139, 157, 169, 185-187
Divine, 78
end of, 66
illusory (banyan) tree, 156
Krishna's words dispel Arjuna's, 115
produced from anger, 26
results in forgetfulness, 26
of separation, 67
soul's capacity to choose, 164
spell of, 193
Impersonal
(contemplation), 127, 128, 129
aspect of God, 132
Indra, 100, 109
Infinite forms, 109
Intelligence, 38, 39, 40, 54, 55, 65, 77, 130, 139, 183
'absorb your...in me', 128
as chariot driver, 69

clear, 26, 191
destroyed by forgetfulness, 26
free from delusion, 23
Krishna speaks through, 143
of the intelligent, 78
swept away by mind, 26
Intention, 37
Intoxication, 47, 151

J
Japa, 110, 112
Janaka, 34
Jaya and Vijaya, 164
Jesus, 44
Jnana yoga, v, 71, 128
Joy, 52, 58, 66, 93, 130, 138, 188, 189, 198
found in work, xii
none without peace, 26
spiritual, 191
Justice vs. forgiveness, 10

K
Kama, 39, 40
Kapila, 110
Karma, xvii, 33, 41, 50, 80, 102, 175, 184
bonds of, 92
how...works, 46
one who is not bound by, 47
relief from the weight of, 106
ropes of, 20
shapes our future, 157
Karma yoga, xv, 29, 59, 71, 129, 191
Karna, 5, 119
Kashiraja, 4
Killing interferes with another's destiny, 18

Index

King of Kashi (Varanasi),
6
Knowledge, 49, 54, 62, 77,
105, 145, 160, 164, 177,
184, 189
and action belong side
by side, 31
is better than practice
(of yoga), 129
comes from Krishna,
160
as greatest gift to others,
177
education (Krishna is),
111
end of, 140, 141
eye of, 158
gift of, 50
goal of, 118
highest of all, 147, 191
is the key, 51
king of, 94
meditation is better
than, 129
most confidential, 92
most secret of all
secrets, 194
of the self, 111
the sum of all, 139
symptoms of self-..., 24,
three kinds of, 184
result of work in spirit
of service, 31
the weapon of, 51
Kripa (Acharya), 5
Krishna, i-vi, 3, 4, 7, 9,
11, 41, 42, 46, 48, 49,
53, 54, 62, 66, 68-70, 75,
80, 82, 83, 86, 90-93, 99,
102, 106, 107, 114, 120,
124-127, 129, 132, 146,

148, 157, 158, 162, 165,
166, 170, 172, 181, 189,
191, 194-196, 197, 198
abode of (Goloka
Vrindavan), 108
is abode, 98
of everlasting truth,
happiness, 154
above even the
enternal, 161
accepts leaf, flower,
fruit, water, 101
accompanies the soul,
17, 44,
and his friends are
ageless, 158
is all, 98
beautiful cowherd boy,
195
all beings are in..., but...
is not in them, 94
all-devouring death, 111
allows illusion to teach
us who we are, xiv
all-pervading, 108
Ancient One, 119
is ancient, 85
appears to protect
religion, 43
as Arjuna's chariot
driver, 8
beginningless, 105
beyond all, 121
beyond senses, 140
beyond darkness, 85,
141
cause of all, 121
chastises Arjuna, 12
is consciousness, 109
as controller, 59
is controlled by Radha's

love, 99
dances with his lovers,
195
is death, 98
descends to earth, 97
destroyer of worlds, 120
is detached, 95
dispeller of doubt, 69
does not interfere, 8, 37,
95
in our freedom, 96
does not want our
forced obedience, 97
drives away darkness,
104
dwells in the heart of all
beings, 193
enduring guardian of
truth, 118
enjoyer of all sacrifices,
100
encourages selfless
work, 61
end of knowledge, 140
equal to all, 102
eternal Personality of
Godhead, 118
eternal seed, 98
is eternal, original,
divine person, 108
exists forever, 78
exists outside all beings,
140
far yet near, 140
is father, 98, 123
favours none, 102
is fire, 98
('s) final message, 195
is flower-bearing spring,
111
('s) form is childlike, 158

friend of every creature, 56, 123
dearmost, 98
gambling of cheats, 111
gives divine wisdom, 104
give everything to, 101
gives heat and rain, 98
gives understanding to come to him, 107
is generous, 96
great souls worship, 96
is goal, 98
of knowledge, 141
God of gods, 108, 121
grandfather of all creatures, 122
heart of...'s message, 190
is hidden, 81, 94
honors our freedom, 8
is immortality, 98
the imperishable, 86
as inexhaustible time, 111
as Infallible One, 7, 122
('s) infinite energies, 116
innermost friend, 59
of inconceivable form, 85
knower of all, 85
is knowledge, 141
knows past, present and future, 17, 81
lets us choose, xvii,
as light of all that shines, 141
as light of the sun and moon, 77, 85
('s) limitless form pervades the cosmos,

121
Lord of lords, 116, 119
Lord of the Universe, 108
Lord of Yoga, 197, 198
lotus-eyed One, 115
('s) love for us, xvi,
as lover, 123
loves all unconditionally, 103
is master, 98
monarch among men, 110
is moon, 160
is morality, 112
('s) nature, 94
is unlimited, 96
is neutral, 7
never leaves Goloka Vrindavan, 158
as ocean, 110
offer...everything, 101
Oldest Person, 121
is Om, 98
is origin, 98, 104
original creator of Brahma, 121
original Godhead, 121
no one knows, 81
as origin of all beings, 96, 105
as origin of the entire universe, 77
all humans would follow...'s path, 34,
perfectly maintains this world, 96
('s) play on earth, 123
plays his flute, 195
poem of his infinite forms, 104

('s) presence felt by those who love him, 103
as prince of the Yadu dynasty, xvii
preserves the devoted, 100
promises to, fulfil our desires, 103
protect devotees, 101
protects the good, 43, 100
is purifier, 98
radiant like the sun, 85
recognizes three classes of faith, 174
refuge, 98, 122
regarded by some as mythological, vii
remembers everything, 43, 44
responds to our desires, xv,
resting place, 98
the ruler, 85
as root of all existence, 23
seated in the hearts of all beings, 109, 160
seed-giving father, 147
shelter of the universe, 121
silent helper and protector, 44
sings the Song of God, xi
smaller than the smallest, 85
smiles, 13
speaks in dreams, 143
source of all, xvi,

Index

source of senses, 140
support of everything, 85
supreme artist, 113
Supreme Goal, 130
Supreme Mystic, 108
supreme shelter of the universe, 118
Supreme Spirit, 108
sustainer, 98
teaches,
    abandon all selfish desires, 28
    all yogas conclude in Bhakti, xvi
    different forms of yoga, 76
    end to suffering, 7
    final assurance (fearlessness), xvi,
    never lament, 18
    three paths of yoga, xv
    is Time, 120
    thousand-armed Cosmic Lord, 123
    is thunderbolt, 110
    transcends qualities of nature, 140
    is wisdom, 112
    is within and beyond everything, 94
    ('s) words never sentimental, 18
    is unborn, 105, 108
    as unseen friend, 8
    is Vedic hymns, 98
    ('s) weapons, 116, 118
    even...works, 34
Krishna consciousness, 59, 86, 93, 96, 195
    brings us from fear to

love, 195
Kshatriya, 190
Kumara brothers, 106
Kuntibhoja, 5
Kuru army, 4, 5, 7
Kurukshetra, iv, 4,
Kusha grass, 64
Kuvera, 110
L
Lamentation, 18
Liberation, 37, 48, 50, 53, 88, 101, 129, 178
    from death, 145
Lion, 110
Lotus, 52, 54
Love,
    eternal spiritual exchange of, 194
    'every living being', 197
    how to...Krishna, 197
    seeing with the eyes of, 123
    as ultimate, xii
M
Magasirsha (month of), 111
Mahabharata, xiii, xiv, 145, 198
Mala, 112
Mantra, 49, 178
Manu(s), 42, 105, 106
Marichi, 109
Maruts, 115, 118
Maya, 79, 159, 193, 194
Meat-eating, 47
Meditation, xiii, 40, 49, 59, 61, 65, 71, 112, 126, 127, 129, 130, 132, 143, 192
    (as superior to knowledge), 129
Mercy (grace), 71, 101,

145, 167, 179, 189, 193, 198
    beyond attraction and aversion, 26
    devotional path depends on, 128
    ends all miseries, 26
    removes all obstacles, 107
Meru, 110
Mind, 22, 24, 38, 39, 40, 44, 54, 55, 64, 65, 77, 82, 130, 139, 151, 158, 187
    absorbed in Krishna, 107
    Arjuna's...full of fear, 122
    controlled, 191
    dies a little every moment, 87
    dwelling on objects sweeps away intelligence, 26
    enemy if uncontrolled, 62
    even of the wise can carry him away, 25,
    'fix your...on me', 128
    foundation of yoga is control of, 63
    friend if subdued, 62
    Krishna speaks through, 143
    limits of human, 116
    organs of, 138
    under control of intelligence, 69
    unsteady...has no peace, 26
    yoga seems unendurable for restless,

68
Misery,
sources of, 57
irony of, 94, 97
Meditation, 40
Merton, Thomas, xiii
Modesty, 139, 164
Moon, 99, 118, 122, 157
"...among stars I am
the...", 109
bright phase of, 89
dark phase, 90
reflects the light of sun,
160
('s) splendor is
Krishna's, 160
Monists, 98
Mundaka Upanishad, 143
Mystic, 60, 67
Krishna is supreme, 109
Krishna's...power
awards vision, 123
lives with Krishna
always, 67
Lord of...Powers, 115,
116
opulences of Krishna,
95, 109, 115
perfect, 67
worships Krishna with
love, 67
N
Nakula, 6
Narada, 108, 110
Narayana, 125
Nature, 84, 85, 142, 152,
153, 156
all are forced to act
according to, 30
binds us, 148
children of, 147

('s) consequences,
divine...leads to Godly
journey, 165
does everything, 35, 55,
144, 145
of the field, 138
impregnated by glance
of Lord, 147
('s) laws, 99
material, 194
Mother, 147
of a person leads to
quality of faith, 173
provides for all her
children, 150
qualities of, 140, 154,
165, 189
three qualities of, 146,
148, 149
soul should be neutral
to, 170
the...of the soul is to
give, 31
of the soul, 138
all souls helpless in...'s
embrace, 95
spell of, 158
spiritual, 48
is womb, 147
Night,
Brahma's, 88
time of awakening for
wise, 27
Nirvana, 64, 66
Non-violence, 139
O
Occupation, 37, 87, 129,
180, 189, 190
Om, 77, 86, 178
Krishna is, 98, 110
Om Tat Sat, 178

Outcaste, 56
P
Panchajanya, 6
Pandavas, 4, 5,
Pandu, 111
the sons of, 4, 6
Paradise,
beyond the rewards of,
21, 22,
souls return to earth
after enjoying, 22
Paramatma (see
Supersoul)
Passion (raja guna), 149,
151, 153, 181, 184-186
charity in, 177
creates need for sexual
partner, 150
faith in, 173
quality of, xv, 78, 79,
148, 170
sacrifice in, 175
Patanjali, 49, 59
Path, 39, 44, 46, 79, 86,
128, 130, 132, 179
abandon other...s, 180
all beings follow
Krishna's, 44
all paths lead to Krishna,
80, 132
best to follow one's
own, 37
binds to work, 149
the contemplative vs.
active, 53, 143
to freedom, 144, 182
of the imperceptible is
difficult, 127
impersonal, 129
of knowledge, 30
Krishna created the

Index

many, 45
of personal devotion, 126
no religious...
  condemned in Gita, 100
of no return, 90
two paths of faith, 30, 43
the right path, 30, 103
of service, 30
of spiritual self-development, 160
of surrender, 131
to transcendence, 69
walk the...given to you, 37
of yoga, 28, 30
Paundra, 5
Peace, 50, 55, 58, 65, 88, 102, 129, 145, 150, 153, 171, 176
all the gods cry, 118
from detachment comes, 129
inner, 34, 187
never found with endless desire, 21
no joy without, 26
found by those without desire, 27
found in the presence of God, 28
ultimate, 193
Peepal (tree), 110, 112
Penance, 48, 70, 78, 90, 106, 124, 132, 173, 174, 176, 177, 178, 181, 189, 192
brings illumination and happiness, 177
human life is meant for,

177
of mind is peacefulness, 176
Perfected beings, 118
Prahlada, 110
Prasadam, 101
Prema, divine love, basis of all emotion, 39, 40
Priests, 103, 110, 178
Purujit, 5

R
Radha (divine mother), 99
  without...Krishna does nothing, 99
Raja guna (see passion), 149
Raja-vidya, 94
Rakshashas, 110
Rama, 111
Reincarnation, 14, 17, 159
  medical science describes, 15
  space between lives, 165
Religion, 71, 132
  abandon all kinds of, 195
  world's...s agree, 171
  beyond conventions of, 70
  essence of, 97
  goal of, 176
  perfection of, 93
  show of, 168
  various practices according to nature, 79
Remembering (the Lord), 59, 82, 87, 99, 109, 129, 180
  remembrance comes from Krishna, 160
Renunciation, 30, 53,

61, 101, 164, 181, 182, 191, 192
in goodness, 182
three kinds of, 181
Ritual, 71, 132, 175
rise above, 21, 23
yogi surpasses, 70
Rope (guna), 149
Rudras, 110, 115, 118
S
Sadhyas, 118
Sacrifice, 47, 49, 84, 132, 167, 172, 174, 178
Krishna is the...of japa, 110
Krishna the real enjoyer of, 58, 100
Krishna rewards all, 82
life without, 177
sense gratification for real freedom, 27
three kinds of, 175
for Vishnu or work binds, 31
wheel of...benefits all, 29
liberates, 31
rain depends on, 99
without attachment, 176
Sages, 117, 138, 148
Sahadeva, 5
Saintly rulers, 103
Samadhi, 24
Samsara, 87, 88
Sankhya, 139
Sattva guna (see goodness), 149
Saumyam, 125
Sanjaya, 4, 7, 11, 121, 125, 197, 198

Index

Sanskrit, xii, xvii, 33, 112,
141, 149
Sat-chit-ananda, 77
Satyaki, 5
Secret, 105, 123
greatest, of all secrets,
93, 194
final, 196
greatest of all, 195
innermost (spiritual),
93, 115
of life, 93, 94
must not be spoken to,
196
Scripture, 20, 21, 89, 22,
33, 49, 51, 89, 145, 169,
170, 173, 175, 176, 179,
187
Seed verses, xvi
Self (see Soul), 39
immortal...as intimate
companion of God, 87
self-hatred, 168
self of the self, 36,
self-torture, 176
self-understanding, 18,
23, 58
transcendent, 39, 144
Selfish motivation, 61
Self-purification, 54
Senses, 35, 37, 38, 39, 54,
58, 86, 127, 129, 139,
159, 183, 186
addicted to...enjoyment,
168
to aid self-discovery, 142
banyan shoots are, 156
control of...purifies the
heart, 64
eleven, 138
give...into the fire, 48

inward control,
outward detachment,
30
make good servants;
bad masters, 26
must be restrained like
sick patient, 26
outward show of...
control, 30
pleasure of the...are a
source of misery, 57
the power of, 25,
the source of, 141
surrender to...pleasures,
166
of touch, etc., 158
transcendental, 65
Serpents (divine), 117
Service,
devotional, 87
to God satisfies the soul,
28
training mind leads to,
63
Seven great enlightened
ones (sages), 105, 106
Sex, 57, 58, 170
promiscuous, 47
partners, 150
Shaibya, 5
Shame, 19, 106
Shankara, iii
Shikhandi, 5
Shark, 111
Shiva, 110, 117
Srila Prabhupada, xvii,
xviii, 197
Sin, 19, 38, 46, 50, 58,
63, 190
force that bind us to,
106

released from all, 105,
195
Skanda, 110
Somadatta, 5
Soma juice, 99
Soul, 142, 150, 151
can be covered by
demoniac mantle, 164
cannot give up work,
182
as child of God, 28
as child of nature, 147
as companion to God,
18, 87
as eternal spirit self, xv,
11, 13, 14, 15, 28, 88, 94,
138, 139, 148
exchanges bodies like
clothing, 16
as forever active, 94
as fragment of God, 17,
159
imperishable, 16
('s) journey, 158
as misunderstood, 18
neither slain nor slayer,
16
never separated, 141
one yet different with
Krishna, 77
pervades body, 16
reincarnates from body
to body, v, 15
seeks pleasure, 33, 142
is small and may forget,
141
as wonderful, 18
wishes to forget utterly,
169
yearns for the presence
of God, 28

Index

Spirit (see Soul)
Spirits, 118, 172
  of the departed, 173
Srila Prabhupada
  Bhaktivedanta means,
  xvii
  encouraged followers to
  write, xvii
Sudra, 190
Suffering, 7, 23, 26, 32, 59,
  65, 103, 142, 177
  can be ended, 13
  companion to illusion,
  13
Sun, 99, 118, 157, 160
  travels north, 90
  travels south, 90
  witness, 139
Supersoul (Paramatma),
  51, 53, 55, 59, 63, 67,
  141, 142, 160, 184
  controls body via
  nature, 145
  dwells within all living
  beings, 137, 144
  enjoyer, 142
  hear the voice of, 159
  Krishna is...in person,
  143
  ordainer, 142
  recognize the.. within
  and in all, 179
  sanction of, 183
  sustainer, 142
  voice of, 187
  Witness, 142
Supreme Person, 155,
  156, 160, 161
Surrender, 22, 94, 131,
  154, 156, 192, 193, 198
Suryavamsa, 41

T
Teacher, 14, 129, 176, 198
  as guides sent by
  Krishna, 71
  Krishna speaks through,
  143
  has seen the truth, 50
  supreme, 122
  wandering...visits king
  (story), 153
Thoreau, Henry David, iii
Three modes, 78
Time, 120
Trance, 65
Transcendence, 56, 69
  above earthly qualities,
  151
Trust, xii, 93, 94, 97, 98,
  102, 178
Truth, 12, 13, 14, 35, 43,
  50, 65, 107, 108, 131,
  140, 162
  discover...where it is
  hard to see, 179
  as eternal, 16
  hardly anyone knows
  Krishna in, 76
  no...found in demoniac,
  165
U
Uccaihshrava, 110
  seekers of, 78
Upanishads, xiii, 22, 69,
  141
Universal Form, xvi, 85,
  96, 112, 114, 116, 117,
  125
Ushana, 111
Uttamauja, son of
  Subhadra, 4, 5
V

Vaishya, 190
Varuna, 110
Vasudeva, 111
Vasuki, 110
Vasus, 110, 115, 118
Vedas, xiii, 22, 32, 33,
  49, 77, 86, 90, 99, 109,
  138, 178
  followers of...seek
  pleasure, 100
  Krishna cannot be seen
  by study of, 124
  Krishna celebrated in
  the, 161
  Rig, Sama, Yajur, 98
  sacred hymns, 156
Vegetarian, 101, 175
Veil
  of desire (covering
  knowledge), 38
  of illusion, 12
  is lifted, 117
  of oblivion (God covers
  soul), 165
Victory, 19, 111, 112
Vikarna, 5
Virata, 5, 6
Vishnu, 109, 119, 164
Vishves, 118
Vivasvan (sun god), 41, 42
Vrindavana, 125, 195
Vrishni, 111
Vyasa, 108, 111, 197, 198
  author of Gita and
  Mahabharata, 198
W
War
  arises in each
  generation, 7
  like a forest fire, 7
Warrior(s), xiv, 3, 14, 19,

who die fighting for justice, 20
Welfare of all, 34
Wilkins, Charles, xiii
Will of God, 28
Wind (like Krishna), 95
spirit (Marichi), 109
'of purifiers I am the...', 111
Wise, 46, 50, 79, 138, 181, 182
act according to their nature, 37
always devoted to Krishna, 97
beyond good and evil, 24
control senses, 26
don't disturb the minds of ignorant, 35
don't lament, 14
focus on Krishna, 25
Krishna is wisdom among the, 112
let go the results of action, 23
serve the Lord with love, 23, 106
withdraw senses as tortoise, 25
Women (qualities of), 111
Work, 46, 47, 51, 53, 55, 61, 129, 166, 191
attachment to...binds self, 148
brings happiness, 31
(s) of charity, sacrifice, penance never given up, 181
does not affect Krishna, 45

done in illusion, 185
God's...sets our pattern, 35
is divine, 47
for Krishna satisfies the whole, 62
renouncing the results of, 181
soul labors to enjoy the fruits of, 139
survival depends on, 32
without...one cannot maintain, 30
without attachment attains Supreme, 33,
to the fruits of action, 128
World Tree (see Banyan), 155, 156, 157
Worship, 12, 61, 67, 80, 96, 97, 98, 99, 100, 100, 101, 103, 122, 124, 125, 127, 143, 145, 161, 173, 175, 176, 179, 190, 190, 195, 196
Y
Yakshas, 110
Yoga, vii, 42, 43, 53, 60, 61, 64, 66, 69, 76, 85, 86, 127, 159, 187
as the art of work, v, 22, 23, 41
different forms of, 76
full absorption in, 105
goal of, 66
as key to happiness, 23
as living in awareness of God, 23
the most perfect in, 127, 128
means undisturbed by

religion, 24
as only way to end birth and death, 88
one in...sees earth, stone, gold as same, 62
as path to freedom, 11,
pure, 90
reach Krishna by regular practice of, 128
supreme secrets of, 197
of renunciation, 101
union with God, 61
waters the root of existence, 54
Yogamaya, 194
Yadu dynasty, xvii
Yudhamanyu, 5
Yudhishthira, 6
Yuyudhana, 5

Ranchor Prime lived in ashrams in Britain and India before working for 20 years as an environmental project manager for the World Wide Fund for Nature and advisor to the Alliance of Religions and Conservation.

other titles by Ranchor Prime:
Hinduism and Ecology
Ramayana: A Journey
Vedic Ecology
Prince of Dharma: the Buddha
Mahavira: Prince of Peace
Hinduism
Cows and the Earth
When the Sun Shines
Birth of Kirtan
The Eight Elements

Charles Newington is a painter, printmaker and illustrator, well known as the creator of The White Horse of Folkestone, a giant hill figure above the Channel Tunnel entrance.
www.charlesnewington.com

MANDALA

An Imprint of MandalaEarth
PO Box 3088
San Rafael, CA 94912
www.MandalaEarth.com

Find us on Facebook: www.facebook.com/MandalaEarth
Follow us on Twitter: @MandalaEarth

First published as *The Illustrated Bhagavad Gita* by Godsfield Press 2003
Text copyright © Ranchor Prime 2003, 2010
Illustrations copyright © Charles Newington 2010

Library of Congress Cataloging-in-Publication Data available.
ISBN: 978-1-64722-470-7

Publisher: Raoul Goff
Associate Publisher: Phillip Jones
VP of Manufacturing: Alix Nicholaeff
Associate Art Director: Ashley Quackenbush
Editorial Director: Katie Killebrew
Editor: Matt Wise
Editorial Assistant: Sophia Wright
Senior Production Manager: Greg Steffen

ROOTS of PEACE   REPLANTED PAPER

Mandala Publishing, in association with Roots of Peace, will plant two trees for each tree used in
the manufacturing of this book. Roots of Peace is an internationally renowned humanitarian
organization dedicated to eradicating land mines worldwide and converting war-torn lands into
productive farms and wildlife habitats. Roots of Peace will plant two million fruit and nut trees in
Afghanistan and provide farmers there with the skills and support necessary for sustainable land use.

Manufactured in India by Insight Editions

10 9 8 7 6 5 4 3 2